BEAT DEPRESSION TO STAY HEALTHIER AND LIVE LONGER

A Guide for Older Adults and Their Families

Gary S. Moak, MD

ROWMAN & LITTLEFIELD
Lanham • Boulder • New York • London

This book represents reference material only. It is not intended as a medical manual, and the data presented here are meant to assist the reader in making informed choices regarding wellness. This book is not a replacement for treatment(s) that the reader's personal physician may have suggested. If the reader believes he or she is experiencing a medical issue, professional medical help is recommended. Mention of particular products, companies, or authorities in this book does not entail endorsement by the publisher or author.

Published by Rowman & Littlefield
A wholly owned subsidiary of
The Rowman & Littlefield Publishing Group, Inc.
4501 Forbes Boulevard, Suite 200, Lanham, Maryland 20706
www.rowman.com

Unit A, Whitacre Mews, 26-34 Stannary Street, London SE11 4AB, United Kingdom

British Library Cataloguing in Publication Information Available

Library of Congress Cataloging-in-Publication Data
Moak, Gary S.
Beat depression to stay healthier and live longer : a guide for older adults and their families / Gary S. Moak, MD.
pages cm
Includes bibliographical references and index.
ISBN 978-1-4422-4661-4 (cloth : alk. paper) — ISBN 978-1-4422-4662-1 (electronic)
1. Depression in old age—Treatment. I. Title.
RC537.5.M63 2016
618.97'68527—dc23
2015031861

♾ ™ The paper used in this publication meets the minimum requirements of American National Standard for Information Sciences Permanence of Paper for Printed Library Materials, ANSI/NISO Z39.48-1992.

Printed in the United States of America

Dedicated to Cheryl Moak, wife, best friend, and partner, without whose love, support, and encouragement this book would not have been possible.

I would like to acknowledge my very dear friend, Dr. Joseph Annibali, for his inspiration and encouragement to write the book and for his excellent reviews of earlier drafts.

CONTENTS

PREFACE

If you've picked up this book, maybe you already realize that depression in old age is a serious problem, one that can spoil the golden years, turning a happy time of life into one of sadness, misery, worry, and despair. Well, it's a bigger problem than you thought. What you may not know is that depression is not just an emotional problem. Left untreated, depression takes a heavy toll on physical health, leading to greater illness, physical disability, and premature death. I refer to this bleak picture as the spiraling decline of depression. It is an untold story and the reason that I wrote *Beat Depression to Stay Healthier and Live Longer: A Guide for Older Adults and Their Families*. This book will not only alert you about the connection between depression and your health, or that of an older adult you care about. It also will tell you what you can do about it.

The good news is that the spiraling decline of depression is preventable, since late-life depression is treatable. Tragically, the vast majority of older adults with depression do not receive treatment for it. They miss their chance to avoid both the suffering of depression and the terrible damage it does to their health. And their friends and family suffer needlessly too, watching them go downhill mentally and physically, while standing by helplessly.

This doesn't have to happen. So why does it? The answer is complicated, but it comes down to two main reasons. First, many older adults with depression deny having a mental health problem, or they decline help that, to them, "smacks" of mental health care. And second, those who are willing to accept help too often have difficulty finding good treatment. Maybe you find this shocking, or maybe you have already come face-to-face with these issues yourself.

Fortunately, you needn't feel helpless or hopeless about depression, regardless of your age or that of the person with depression you care about. *Beat Depression to Stay Healthier and Live Longer* will help you deal with depression. Reading this book, you will see that depression is not simply an expectable reaction to being old but a real brain disease that can be diagnosed and treated. You will learn how to identify the various forms of depression and to recognize other conditions that masquerade as depression. Most important, you will learn how depression can worsen diseases such as diabetes, chronic lung disease, heart failure, chronic kidney disease, arthritis, and cancer, and how it can increase the chance of heart attack, stroke, Alzheimer's disease, Parkinson's disease, and dying prematurely. You will learn about treatment of depression in older adults and find out how to recognize good treatment and find it. You will see that depression is treatable—you can get your life back! And finally, you will find advice about how to help a reluctant elder accept professional help, whether it's for yourself or someone you care about. I hope this will help you feel more confident about seeking treatment for depression or encouraging someone you care about to do so.

All the older adults I know worry about Alzheimer's disease to one degree or another. In my opinion, depression is just as big a threat to the golden years. My patients with depression seem to suffer more than those with Alzheimer's disease. And depression leads to worsening health, disability, and premature death, whereas Alzheimer's disease does not. Depression is also more common than Alzheimer's disease. Our best estimates are that clinically significant depression affects one in five older adults. Among certain groups of older adults, it is even more common. Depression affects 40 percent of nursing home residents, 40 percent of those with Alzheimer's disease, and half of those with Parkinson's disease. And at least half of all caregivers of persons with dementia have depression.

Depression doesn't affect only the person who has it. I consider depression in old age to be a family illness. It disrupts family life and is very stressful for family members. In fact, depression is disruptive to us all. According to the World Health Organization, depression is the second leading cause of disability around the world. And it quadruples the cost of all health care, which, these days, no society can afford.

I wrote *Beat Depression to Stay Healthier and Live Longer* based on my thirty years of experience practicing geriatric psychiatry and working with older patients and their families. Each day, I spend much of my time talking with patients and their family members about normal aging, late-life depression, and treatment.

By the time patients find their way to my practice, many are frustrated and desperate for help. They are lost and do not know where to turn. Some have sought answers to their questions on the Internet but found the information confusing or not applicable to older adults. Very early in my career I realized that successful treatment of older patients depended upon teaching them and their family members about depression and its treatment. In my daily practice I answer the questions my patients and their family members ask. I also make them aware of things they did not know they needed to know. My patients and their family members express relief that they've come to the right place and found a doctor they can talk to and understand! I want my readers to share that same feeling.

Over the years, I have extended my efforts to educate older adults and family members about late-life depression to roles outside of my one-on-one practice with patients. After completing my own training in geriatric psychiatry in 1986, I joined the faculty at the University of Massachusetts Medical School, where I taught for twenty-nine years before joining the faculty of the Geisel Medical School at Dartmouth. Over the years, I have enjoyed teaching doctors-in-training about aging and mental health.

I also spent many years working on educational projects for the American Association for Geriatric Psychiatry. As chairman of the Clinical Practice Committee, member of the board of directors, secretary-treasurer, and president, I worked on educational initiatives for the public and healthcare professionals alike. The goals of these projects were to improve public understanding about aging and depression, and to combat the stigma of aging and mental illness. This book is a natural extension of all these efforts.

If you are an older adult with depression, then *Beat Depression to Stay Healthier and Live Longer* is written for you. If you are worried about an older adult with depression and wondering what you can do to help, then this book is for you too. I wrote this book in the same way I talk to patients and their family members. In a way, they helped me write the book, since much of the content comes from their questions and the answers I gave them that they found helpful.

The information in this book is practical and will answer many questions you have. It will lead you to think differently about depression and tip you off about things you didn't know you needed to know. It will help you to ask your doctor the right questions so you can get the help you need to get your life back.

Throughout *Beat Depression to Stay Healthier and Live Longer*, I use case stories to illustrate the points I make. These stories are snippets or composites of case histories of patients whom I treated. I have changed the names and many of the details to protect their privacy and confidentiality. My patients are usually glad to let me use their stories to help others. Some even like to help with the storytelling personally: over the years, many have proudly participated in my various teaching activities with medical students and residents.

You can use this book in different ways to learn what you need to know. Obviously, the book can be read in its entirety from cover to cover. I think you will find it worthwhile to take the time to read it this way. Some readers, however, may prefer to use the book as a reference, reading only those chapters of immediate interest. I organized it with this in mind.

The book is divided into three sections. Part 1 contains chapters intended to help you get a better understanding of depression in the elderly. Part 2 consists of chapters each covering the impact depression has on a physical disease (e.g., diabetes), group of diseases (e.g., cardiovascular disease), or type of geriatric problem (e.g., falling). You might decide, for example, to read just the chapters on depression and heart disease or depression and diabetes, and skip the others in this section for now. Finally, the chapters in part 3 will tell you about treatment for depression in late life, suggest things you can do for yourself, and coach you about working with professionals in the healthcare system to get help.

However you make use of this book, please keep in mind that medicine is not an exact science, and geriatric psychiatry is one of medicine's more complicated specialties. I based this book on my own professional experience and the most cutting-edge scientific knowledge at the time I wrote it. As you read it, please keep in mind that medical science constantly changes, and what applies on average may not be right for you. Please do not use this book to make decisions on your own about your health. Instead use it as a guide to working with healthcare professionals to get the help you need.

Finally, I offer a few words about some of the terms I use. Throughout the book, I will refer to the elderly in various ways, including "older adults," "seniors," "elders," and "geriatric patients." I will also use the terms "elderly" and "old age." Many writers avoid "elderly" and "old age" as if these terms are offensive. I think this type of thinking is wrong. Avoiding terms such as "old age" and "the elderly" furthers stigma and negative attitudes. We need to stop treating old age as a taboo subject. It's not. With any luck, we'll all get there. Old age doesn't have to be something awful, to dread. For many, it turns out to be their happiest time of life.

Thus I will use all of these terms throughout the book. I prefer "older adults" because there is no "the" as in "the elderly." The "the" lumps together all old people as if they are somehow all the same. They are not. Older adults are more varied than any other age group. "Older adults," on the other hand, suggests a wide collection of unique individuals over age fifty-five. I wrote this book for people in their seventies, eighties, nineties, and beyond, and those slightly younger adults who will be there soon.

I hope that reading this book helps you to address depression and find effective treatment. If you do, and if you get your life back, then I'll be as pleased as if I treated you myself.

DEPRESSION IS A LIFE AND DEATH MATTER

A Tale of Two Sydneys

For two retired salesmen, Sydney Allen and Sydney Brown (we'll call them Sydney A and Sydney B), retirement was the best of times . . . until it wasn't. At age eighty-two, each had a stroke, and suddenly everything changed. Each man felt as if the rug had been pulled out from under him. For Sydney A, things were eventually okay. He recovered. For Sydney B, they weren't. His health went from bad to worse. The rest of his life was the worst of times. The difference was depression and the toll it took.

Stroke led to the occurrence, in each Sydney, of a type of depression called post-stroke depression. Both experienced it as a fairly dark depression. Each felt as if he had fallen into a black hole of gloom and despair from which there was no escape.

Sydney A had treatment for his depression. It took some doing, but his family convinced him to start the treatment and stick with it. His depression cleared up, he recovered from his stroke, and resumed most of his activities. He got his life back and lived another ten years.

Sydney B didn't have treatment for depression. He stubbornly declined any professional help, and his family went along with this decision, viewing it as a natural and understandable reaction to the circumstances. Sydney B remained depressed and never recovered from his stroke. Depression caused his health to deteriorate faster, and he died after four miserable years.

This tale of two Sydneys is a story not only about the mental anguish of depression but also about how depression can ruin health and bring about premature death. It is a cautionary tale.

The Sydneys had much in common until depression steered them down different paths. Both men had been successful salesmen and family men. Sydney A sold plumbing supplies, and Sydney B sold insurance. Each had retired at age seventy, at the top of his game. Both Sydneys served in the military during the Vietnam conflict. Each was posted stateside, and neither saw combat. Sydney A married the sister of a friend he met during his service in the army. Sydney B married his high school sweetheart.

Retirement had been great for both Sydneys. Each had been a confident, self-assured individual, happily married, still living independently in his home, financially secure, and in good health. Children and grandchildren lived nearby, family life was good, and both were physically vigorous. They enjoyed golf, tennis, bicycling, and travel.

The strokes came out of the blue and caused similar symptoms, which included right-side weakness and difficulty walking and speaking. After several days in the hospital, both Sydneys were sent to rehabilitation facilities. Initially things went as expected. Of course, there were the normal emotional reactions: dismay about having a stroke, apprehension about the future, and frustration, particularly over difficulty speaking. But each was determined to recover, and the doctors seemed pleased with their progress.

Then depression set in. As we will see in chapter 3, post-stroke depression commonly occurs after a stroke. This type of depression can be very severe, and it can interfere with recovery. The symptoms of depression Sydney A and Sydney B experienced were very similar. Foremost was profound sadness that tenaciously enshrouded them day in and day out. There were periods of crying, pessimistic and hopeless thinking, all-consuming fretful worries, and despair, during which they felt convinced they would be better off dead. The crying was particularly hard for family members because no one had ever seen either man cry. Each had always been the family rock.

There were also bodily symptoms. Both men had complete loss of appetite. Food had no appeal, and they each lost about fifteen pounds.

There was terrible insomnia. Falling asleep was no trouble, but between two and four o'clock, they would wake up and lie awake for the rest of the night in a state of dread. Both men complained of lack of energy and motivation, and neither made much effort in rehabilitation therapies.

Psychiatrists call this pattern of depression symptoms major depression. We will learn about the different forms of depression in chapter 4. For now, suffice it to say, major depression is a serious condition that, as we will soon see, can lead to deteriorating health, disability, and premature death.

The doctors became alarmed when the Sydneys began refusing to participate in rehabilitation therapies. Because each felt a terrible, unjustified sense of hopelessness, therapy sessions seemed useless. The gains they initially had made quickly disappeared, and each now seemed worse than right after the stroke. The doctors arranged for consultations with psychiatrists. At this juncture, the Sydneys' destinies diverged.

Sydney B didn't want to see the psychiatrist. He was taken aback by the idea. After all, he wasn't "crazy." He'd always had good mental health, been able to solve his own problems and stand on his own two feet. He didn't need "*that* kind" of help. Seeing a psychiatrist would be embarrassing and humiliating. No—he would handle things himself. And, anyway, what was the point? He thought his situation was hopeless and felt that his life was over. What good would talking to a psychiatrist do? The psychiatrist couldn't repair the damage from the stroke. Sydney B was also afraid that the psychiatrist would have him "put away."

Sydney B's son, Bill, was his father's healthcare proxy. Father and son had been very close over the years. Seeing his father this way left Bill emotionally crushed. What made it so terribly demoralizing for him was that he shared his father's pessimistic views of old age, depression, psychiatrists, and psychiatric treatment. Bill concluded that his father's life was over, for all intents and purposes. He steeled himself to accept that his father would never be the same, stopped wishing for him to recover, and went into a type of mourning. Bill couldn't understand why they would want his father to see a psychiatrist or be treated for depression: "After all he'd been through already, why on earth did they want to put him through that? Why couldn't they leave him alone?" The rehab doctor tried to explain his reasoning, but Bill didn't want any part of it. He rationalized, "Of course my dad's depressed, he had a stroke! Wouldn't you be depressed? It's understandable. He doesn't need psychiatric help for that!"

Time went on, and Sydney B went home. Bill and the rest of the family felt that going home would lift Sydney B's spirits. In fact, Sydney B was glad to go home, but the depression was unrelenting. He remained negative, pessimistic, and unmotivated. He still had no interest in therapy. At the urging of his family, he cooperated reluctantly with the physical therapist, but he made no progress. Mostly he stayed in bed or sat on the couch, feeling sorry for himself and thinking that he was becoming a bigger and bigger burden on his family.

Over the next year, depression caused Sydney B's condition to worsen in three ways. First, due to the inactivity, his muscles got weaker and weaker and eventually started to shrink, a process called deconditioning. This left him feeling insecure, even more useless and helpless, and more depressed. He walked less, and when he did, he was wobbly, unsteady, and afraid of falling. Inevitably, he did fall. And then he fell again and again. Chapter 16 deals entirely with depression as a cause of falling.

With the third fall, Sydney B broke his hip. He was taken to the hospital and underwent surgery to repair the broken bone. The surgery went well, and Sydney B recovered physically without complications. But now everything seemed even more hopeless. He was more depressed and filled with self-pity. He told Bill that if he had a gun he'd shoot himself. Sydney B was again sent to rehab. This time, however, he made no progress at all. He never walked again and had to go live in a nursing home.

The next year in the nursing home was heartbreaking. Sydney B continued to be depressed. He always seemed sad, gloomy, and morose. He mostly stayed in his room, either in bed or sitting in a chair, just staring into space.

Then came Sydney B's next decline in health. He developed diabetes. Because of his debilitation, it was not possible for him to control the diabetes with exercise or other lifestyle changes. Pills were necessary to control his blood sugar. Depression made Sydney B's sugars hard to control. He needed more and more medications, some of which had side effects. Eventually, he had to start taking insulin shots. In chapter 8 we will learn about the two-way street between depression and diabetes.

The nursing home staff prevailed upon Sydney B's son, Bill, to allow a mental health specialist to see his father. Bill relented, but half-heartedly. A psychotherapist, what people often call a counselor, visited Sydney B several times. Sydney B was generally polite, but sessions were like pulling teeth. Sydney B felt the visits were futile, and he had nothing to say. He began to refuse to see the therapist. Bill even agreed to allow the doctor to prescribe an antidepressant medication. However, after one month of treatment, Sydney B was no better. The medication made Sydney B constipated, and Bill said "enough is enough"— and insisted the medication be stopped.

More time went by, and Sydney B started to decline mentally. He became forgetful and confused. He no longer could remember where he was, how to work the remote control for his television, or how to use his cell phone to call his family. Sydney B now had dementia. The stroke, subsequent falls with mild head injuries, uncontrolled diabetes, and depression all had a hand in bringing it on. Over the next six months, Sydney B developed chest pain, fluid retention in his feet and legs, and shortness of breath. Nearly four years after his stroke, Sydney B had a massive heart attack and died.

Sydney A avoided this fate. While he developed as severe a post-stroke depression as Sydney B, and likewise initially turned down treatment, Sydney A eventually did accept treatment, got better, and got his life back. The difference was Sydney A's daughter, Elaine.

Elaine had a hopeful attitude, believing that her father could recover and refusing to accept that his good years were all behind him. She saw the depression as a bigger threat to Sydney A's recovery and well-being than the stroke. You see, Elaine knew a little about depression in the elderly from prior experience. Her mother-in-law had severe depression, but she responded to medical treatment and returned to normal. Elaine was determined not to give up without a fight. She requested that her father be seen by a psychiatrist and was relieved to learn that the psychiatrist thought antidepressant medication was indicated. Sydney A did not want to take the medication, but Elaine patiently encouraged him, and, eventually, he agreed.

Treatment of depression in fragile older adults is often an arduous process. We will see why this is in chapter 21. Sydney A needed Elaine's

constant encouragement to stick with the treatment. Several adjustments of the medication were needed, but after almost eight weeks,
Sydney A started to get better. The crying spells stopped, he became
less negative and pessimistic, and he began to eat better. He resumed
his therapy and actually tried hard. His walking and speech steadily
improved, and a few weeks later he was able to go home.

Returning home lifted Sydney A's spirits further, and he felt encouraged. The more progress he made physically the better his mood got,
and the better his mood got the more progress he made physically.
Sydney A started to enjoy seeing his grandchildren again. His speaking
ability improved little by little. After four months he was walking without a cane, at six months he resumed driving, and at ten months speech
problems were barely noticeable. A full year after his stroke, Sydney A
was back on the golf course. He was not the ten-handicap golfer he
used to be—he had lost twenty strokes on his score—but he was delighted.

Sydney A felt fortunate and optimistic. Despite a stroke, he was still
fully independent. He still lived at home, was able to travel with his
wife, and enjoyed spending time with his grandchildren. He felt well
and was determined to shave ten strokes off his game. He had gotten
his life back.

Over the next three years, Sydney A became prediabetic. Following
the diet and exercise plan his doctor laid out for him, he was able to
control it without medications, at least for a few more years. After that,
a daily pill was all that was needed to keep the diabetes in check.

During the coming years, Sydney A felt happy and content. He took
his psychiatrist's advice and remained on the medication for depression.
He noticed slight forgetfulness and occasional trouble getting his words
to come out. But he never required help managing any of his affairs,
and he did not develop dementia. He was satisfied with his life. A
grandson's wedding and a sixtieth anniversary cruise with his wife were
especially joyful for him. Sydney A lived six years longer than Sydney B.
Despite having had a stroke, Sydney A felt these had been some of the
happiest years of his life.

In chapter 7 we will see that depression increases the chance of
having a stroke. In this tale of two Sydneys, the opposite happened—
stroke caused depression. But then depression made things go from bad
to worse.

Each of the illnesses described in the chapters in part 2 can be as devastating and catastrophic as stroke. As we shall see, depression is a cause of many illnesses. Or, as in the "Tale of Two Sydneys," depression may alter the course of an illness, diverting it from manageable problem to life-changing calamity. What happened to each Sydney had more to do with depression than stroke.

Sydney A had treatment for depression, and he recovered. Sydney B did not have treatment for depression, and he remained depressed. Depression did not just make Sydney B sad, morose, hopeless, and withdrawn. Depression made him weaker and weaker and prone to falling. Eventually he did fall and wound up in a nursing home—all indirectly due to depression. Depression brought on diabetes and made it harder to control. Depression contributed to his becoming demented, making his last years that much more tragic. Depression also increased his risk for heart attack. Eventually he had a heart attack and died. While the cause of death was heart attack, Sydney B died of depression.

Sydney B is not an isolated case. Depression in older adults is often not diagnosed properly or treated effectively. The majority of older adults with depression do not receive treatment for it.[1] The extra suffering, illness, disability, and missed years are horrible to think about. Of course, suicide is the most shocking way in which depression causes death. This has to be taken very seriously by everyone involved with a depressed elder, because elderly people have the highest rate of suicide of any group, especially men over the age of eighty-five. Certainly I do not mean to ignore suicide, but I wrote this book to sound an alarm about how depression brings about premature death through its corrosive effects on health.

Sydney A avoided this fate. He had treatment for depression and got better. This allowed him to recover more fully from the stroke. He got his life back—well, truth be told, not completely. Never again was he able to shoot lower than ninety on the golf course, but he enjoyed the game as much anyway.

Obviously, old age does not always have happy endings. There are many sad and unhappy aspects. In the next few chapters, we'll explore the difference between normal emotional distress and depressive illness, and we will learn to understand the difference between feeling depressed, which can be normal, at times, and having depression, a serious medical illness. Having depression is not a normal part of aging.

In this sense, old age is not depressing. Depression, when present, should not be endured as expectable and normal. Those who allow depression to go unchecked leave themselves in undue peril, without realizing it. Had Sydney B's son, Bill, known this, maybe he would have acted as did Sydney A's daughter, Elaine. He might have advocated for his father to have treatment for depression, and Sydney B might have had a chance to get his life back, too.

Part I

Depression in Late Life: What It Is and What It Is Not

1

OLD AGE IS *NOT* DEPRESSING

Truth and Fiction

Why do older people who have enjoyed good mental health their entire lives become depressed for the first time in old age? The commonsense answer most of us arrive at, based on our own experience, is that old age simply is depressing. Illness, disability, loss of independence, and death all seem depressing, so we assume these cause depression in older adults. But, with the exception of a small number of specialists who know a lot about brain science, most of us have the wrong idea about the causes of depression in old age. I would like you to consider that your beliefs about the causes of depression in old age might be incorrect. In these first few chapters I will ask you to think differently about this serious medical illness in older adults.

Before we go on, let's consider the case of Agnes, a ninety-year-old woman who was forced to move into an assisted living facility after falling made it unsafe for her to remain at home. Agnes had diabetes, congestive heart failure, and arthritis, all of which conspired to make her weaker and frailer. She developed difficulty walking, felt unsteady at times, and became less mobile. After a fall on the stairs, Agnes's children insisted that she sell her house and move into an assisted living facility, near her daughter, in another state.

Several months later I saw Agnes and found her to have moderately severe depression. She told me that she was sad and gloomy all the time, nothing gave her pleasure any longer, and she felt worthless and wanted to die. Based on my assessment, I was confident that I could help Agnes get better, and I recommended treatment to her.

But Agnes had other ideas. She wanted no part of any treatment for depression, explaining, "I'm ninety, in declining health, and I live in assisted living; this is how I'm supposed to feel." Maybe you agree with Agnes that depression seems an understandable and normal reaction to all that has happened to her. You might also be wondering whether anything can or should be done about it at her age.

Fortunately, in time, I was able to persuade Agnes to accept treatment with antidepressant medication, and she responded quite well. Within a few months she felt better. Shortly thereafter, she took up painting, a hobby she'd given up after her children were born. Before long she was teaching art lessons to other residents and became chairperson of the residents' council. You might be surprised to learn that Agnes told me, "This is the best time of my life. I'm enjoying myself in ways I never thought I could." Agnes's daughter was even more emphatic. "Thank you, thank you, thank you," she gushed. "We thought Mom's life was over, but you gave her back to us for a few good years!" I was very touched when Agnes gave me one of her paintings in gratitude for helping her get her life back.

As a geriatric psychiatrist, I treat patients like Agnes every day. I am fortunate to hear such expressions of relief, joy, and gratitude. But that's not always the case. It's not unusual to encounter rejection of my recommendations for treatment. Usually it goes something like this: "Of course Mom's depressed. She just had a stroke. Who wouldn't be depressed? She doesn't need to see a psychiatrist for that! It's normal." Such attitudes and beliefs are ill informed and can have tragic results. They prevent millions of older adults from receiving treatment that can help, instead consigning them to an old age of misery, deteriorating health, and premature death.

Effective treatment for depression in old age has been available since the 1960s, yet in the twenty-first century the majority of older adults with depression still do not receive treatment.[1] They live with depression year after year. The reasons behind this are complicated, but foremost among them are misinformed attitudes in our culture about aging, mental health, and depression. Seniors, and those in a position to help them, too often do not recognize depression as a problem for which medical treatment should be sought. They see depression as an expectable, inevitable, and normal part of aging, for which nothing need be done. And they view psychiatric treatment as a sign of weakness, or believe that the elderly do not get better, so treatment is futile.

If you are still not convinced, don't worry—you are not alone. Part of the problem is that the word "depression" itself is confusing. In day-to-day conversation we use "depression" to describe normal feelings of sadness or gloominess we all have, from time to time. In healthcare settings, medical professionals use "depression" as shorthand for a number of serious medical illnesses causing unhappy mood disturbances. The difference between feelings of depression and depressive illness is apples and oranges, and it is important to keep this in mind.

We all normally feel depressed at different times in our lives when faced with challenging circumstances. These feelings come and go, and subside over time. Most of the time we understand what makes us feel depressed. Naturally, when friends or relatives have a depressive illness, we put two and two together and assume that depressing circumstances must be causing their depression.

This approach helps us understand the normal emotional reactions of healthy people, but it doesn't work so well for those with serious, clinical depression. This type of depression may occur even when life is going well. It may not improve on its own, and it affects daily functioning. In this book we will focus on depressive illness, a serious brain disease. Serious depression in older adults comes about for different reasons than the depression we all feel when depressing things happen. When an elder you care about has severe depression, try not to assume that depressing circumstances they might be dealing with are the cause, because this can be harmful to them in at least three ways.

First, such conclusions reinforce the social stigma associated with depression. Much of the public views depression as a sign of weakness. The belief that depression is an understandable reaction to depressing circumstances implies that a person is depressed because he or she is too weak to cope with those circumstances. Depressed elders who feel ashamed about being depressed may deny they have it, insist they must work it out themselves, or decide just to live with it.

Rosalind, an eighty-four-year-old widow living in a retirement community, was one such patient. She was a retired high school English teacher who had been happily married to a colleague until his death some fifteen years earlier. Rosalind had depression that had been going on for more than a year. The nurse in her building convinced her to see me, and Rosalind allowed the nurse to call my office to make an appointment. Rosalind graciously welcomed me into her apartment—I make house calls—but made it clear that she didn't think she needed my help. She admitted she had depression but "not the real kind of depression . . . just the old-age kind." Older adults harboring such feelings stubbornly ignore the pleas of worried relatives or caregivers to accept medical help.

Second, when elders or their family members view depression as a purely psychological problem, they may not recognize the need for a thorough medical evaluation. Such evaluation may uncover physical causes of depression that need to be corrected.

Third, depression is associated with harmful effects on health and longevity. We'll cover this in detail throughout much of the rest of the book. For now, here are just some of the facts about depression and health that people should know:

- Depression increases the chance of having a stroke.
- After a heart attack, depression doubles the chance of dying.
- Depression makes chronic pain worse and harder to treat. Treatment of depression lessens the severity of chronic pain.
- Depression makes diabetes harder to control.
- Depression makes diseases such as congestive heart failure, arthritis, and Parkinson's disease more disabling.
- Depression increases the likelihood that patients with chronic kidney disease will need to go on dialysis.
- Depression nearly doubles the chance of getting Alzheimer's disease or Parkinson's disease.
- Depression weakens the immune system, making it harder to fight infection.
- Older persons with depression die sooner, from all causes, than those who are not depressed.

Such facts, and many others, constitute an untold story about depression, aging, and health known only to a few specialists. Older persons who ignore depression put their health in jeopardy. I find that when I dispel incorrect notions about depression and help my patients understand that it is a brain disease that can take a serious toll on their health, they become much more receptive to having treatment.

The remainder of this chapter deals with what depression is not. I will dispel a number of commonly held beliefs and misconceptions about mental health and aging that often result in needless suffering in old age. In chapter 2, we will begin to see what depression is and what actually causes it in later life.

FALSE BELIEF 1: MENTAL ILLNESS IS AN INEVITABLE PART OF AGING

The belief that mental illness is just what happens to you when you grow old is surprisingly widespread. Many people assume that "senility," dementia, Alzheimer's disease, depression, "the blues," and "shot nerves" are part of the deal. They firmly believe that becoming mentally impaired, in one way or another, is inevitable in old age.[2]

It is true that mental illness is more common among the elderly but so are arthritis, high blood pressure, diabetes, emphysema, heart disease, and cancer. None of these conditions is inevitable, and we certainly don't consider them "normal"—we accept them as diseases that should be treated. It is striking that, while the majority of older adults have one or more chronic physical illness, the majority do not have mental illness. Only about one in nine has Alzheimer's disease,[3] and one in five has clinically significant depression.[4] These problems are far from inevitable. Yet most of my patients and members of their families are surprised when I tell them that good mental health is the normal expectation in old age.

FALSE BELIEF 2: ALL MENTAL ILLNESS IN OLD AGE IS SENILITY

I still encounter older patients, or members of their families, who believe that all old-age mental health problems, including depression, represent a form of "senility."[5] Many have heard that there is no cure for Alzheimer's disease, which they equate with "senility." This makes them think that nothing can be done for any mental health problem in late life. They conclude that there is no point to seeking help for depression because it does no good and only leads to a bleak existence in a nursing home.

These beliefs are especially harmful and incorrect. All mental illness in old age is not "senility" any more than all cases of diarrhea, constipation, or blood in the stool are colon cancer. It is true that there is no cure for Alzheimer's disease, but there is treatment that can help patients live with it better. And depression is often completely treatable. As we saw with Agnes, older patients with depression can get their lives back.

FALSE BELIEF 3: DEPRESSION AMONG THE ELDERLY IS A NORMAL AND EXPECTED PART OF AGING BECAUSE OLD AGE IS DEPRESSING

To the contrary, while many older adults get depression, it is not because old age itself is depressing. In fact, some studies show that older adults have higher levels of happiness than younger people.[6] This is true even among many of those who live with chronic disease, physical limitations, and activity restrictions.

The elderly are survivors. Many have lived through wars, personal calamities, and family tragedies. Coping with such challenges may have helped them develop resilience and wisdom about life that younger people may not yet possess. Older adults who do not have depression may handle tragedy better than many younger people. It may come as a surprise that some studies of posttraumatic stress disorder show that older adults cope with disaster better than do younger victims.[7]

This is not to say that older adults do not get the blues. Old age can be a difficult time of life, and many trying and sad things happen. Aging confronts us with loss of our youthful appearance and vigor, illness, disability, and the deaths of friends, relatives, and ultimately ourselves. We may come to see ourselves as over the hill or has-beens. Loss of independence and autonomy is a bitter pill to swallow. Unhappiness about these developments is normal, but mentally healthy older adults have the maturity, perspective, and wisdom to cope with such challenges. Old age doesn't make people depressed. It's the other way around: depression keeps elders from coping with old age. Old age itself is not depressing.[8]

FALSE BELIEF 4: BECAUSE DEPRESSION IS "JUST WHAT HAPPENS TO YOU" WHEN YOU GET OLD, NOTHING SHOULD BE DONE ABOUT IT

Agnes shared this common view. The attitude that you must accept depression as "part of the deal" in reaching old age makes little sense when you consider how often those holding this view seek medical treatment for arthritis or undergo cataract surgery or hip replacement. All medical care of older adults is meant to relieve suffering, improve quality of life, prevent further decline of health, and prevent premature death. These goals apply to treatment of depression as much as to any other health problem.

FALSE BELIEF 5: DEPRESSION IS A PROBLEM THAT YOU HAVE TO HANDLE ON YOUR OWN

Eleanor was a seventy-seven-year-old former bookkeeper who raised five children and always "ran a tight ship." She looked shocked when she said to me, "I've always been able to handle my problems. Why can't I handle them now?" This sentiment echoes the consternation many of my patients feel about having depression. Depression has made them feel as if the proverbial rug has been pulled out from under them.

If you've taken good mental health for granted your entire life, it can feel like a type of betrayal to find yourself unable to control your emotions. In our day-to-day lives, we feel in control of our minds. We could not function very well without this feeling. We do not have a similar sensation of control of our other bodily organs, such as the heart, lungs, kidneys, or liver, nor do we expect to. This difference in perception is a big part of why we have a different attitude about mental health problems than other health problems.

One of my patients, an eighty-three-year-old gentleman named Don, once described this bias with an elegant metaphor I've always remembered. He had moderate depression that he'd been living with for almost two years. I thought treatment would help him, but he didn't want any part of it. In explaining his reluctance, he told me he couldn't accept the idea that he wasn't "sailing his own boat." The pills he took for his thyroid, heart, and lungs were okay because "you have no control over those organs." But he saw medical treatment for the mind as different because "you should be able to control it yourself." Such thinking is often behind patients' steadfast insistence that they must pull themselves out of it.

Severe depression is not something people can pull themselves out of any more than they can pull themselves out of congestive heart failure, kidney disease, or gallstones. When patients with congestive heart failure develop difficulty breathing, they are usually grateful for treatment that relieves their distress. They rarely believe they can handle such illnesses themselves because they have no sense of being in control over the workings of their heart. We also do not sense our brains at work, but we feel in control of our minds. This sense of being in control of our minds allows those with depression to believe they can pull themselves out of the severe depression. In my experience, once older adults understand that depression is a disease of the brain, and not something they have control over, they become more open to considering treatment. It's not that they can't handle their problems any longer; rather, their brain has let them down. I often say to my patients, "It's not you; it's your brain." We will talk about the difference between the mind and the brain in the next chapter.

FALSE BELIEF 6: DEPRESSION IS A SIGN OF WEAKNESS

Closely related to the belief that depression is a problem one must handle oneself is the notion that depression is a sign of personal weakness or moral failure. People harboring such sentiments feel even worse about accepting psychiatric treatment. They often believe they wouldn't feel so bad if they were better persons, tried harder, or prayed more. For many, agreeing to psychiatric treatment is a personal disgrace. Others see depression as a cross they must bear stoically.

Older adults usually handle their declining physical strength and deteriorating health without taking these as signs of personal weakness or failure. Some elders even view physical infirmities as badges of honor, as did my patient who saw his frozen shoulders and painful, creaking knees as the price he paid for a productive life supporting his family as a construction worker. Smokers may blame themselves for lung disease, but elderly patients with a wide range of illnesses, from stroke to osteoporosis, usually don't blame themselves.

Many people feel differently about depression, which they see as a malady of the spirit. Marvin, a ninety-two-year-old retired stockbroker, actually described it this way when he told me that depression was "decapitating [his] spirit." Because he saw this as a spiritual problem and not a medical problem, he planned to seek advice from his rabbi. He thought taking antidepressant medication would be cowardly.

FALSE BELIEF 7: TREATMENT FOR DEPRESSION IS USELESS SINCE THE ELDERLY DON'T GET BETTER

One facet of the negative, pessimistic attitudes about old age is the belief that medical treatment is futile because the elderly do not get better. I am always dismayed when patients or members of their families tell me this. Pessimism about treatment is not limited to mental health problems. An older woman with depression and extremely painful arthritis that limited her mobility told me she had never sought treatment for the arthritis believing that nothing could be done to make it better.

Doubts about the value of medical treatment are greatest when it comes to mental disorders, including depression. Now, we must acknowledge that not all geriatric health problems are treatable. But many mental disorders are very treatable, and usually something can be done to improve patients' lives, even for conditions such as Alzheimer's disease, which currently has no cure.

When it comes to late-life depression, the belief that treatment does not work is just plain wrong. Old people with depression do get better. Decades of clinical experience by geriatric psychiatrists worldwide bear this out. My own experience over thirty years, treating thousands of older adults with depression, has shown me that treatment works. And numerous research studies have proven that older adults do respond to treatment for depression, and they do so nearly as well as do younger patients. As we will see in chapter 18, there are many effective options for treating depression in the elderly.

FALSE BELIEF 8: DEPRESSION IS "ALL IN YOUR MIND"

You can see a broken arm on an x-ray, and the cast is a tangible sign of it. Your orthopedic surgeon can show you the arthritis in your hips on your x-rays. The surgeon can see your tumor during the operation to remove it, and the pathologist can see under the microscope what kind of cancer you have. Blood tests provide objective evidence of diabetes and elevated cholesterol. In contrast, until recently, no one has been able to "see" depression. Newer types of brain-imaging technologies are beginning to allow scientists to see the telltale signs of depression in the brain. We'll learn about this in the next chapter. Despite these scientific advances, in the minds of most people depression remains all in the mind, still a purely subjective condition. No tests or biopsies can be done for it, and surgeons can't cut it out.

Because the symptoms of depression are mental and behavioral, it does not seem real to many people. By comparison, even Alzheimer's disease, another late-life mental condition, whose symptoms are mental and behavioral, seems more real. Loss of memory and other cognitive abilities brings about obvious disability. When the phone rings, and you see an older adult with Alzheimer's disease try to answer it using the television remote control, it's pretty obvious that something is terribly wrong with his or her brain.

Depression can be as disabling as Alzheimer's disease, but it can be much harder for patients and family members to understand why they seem so incapable and helpless. Depressed patients still know how to do things; they simple don't do them. People with Alzheimer's disease may not know how to dress themselves any longer. Some of those with depression may not be able to dress themselves either. Not because they no longer know how but because it feels like too daunting a task to face. It is hard for observers to understand this.

The helpless and dependent behaviors of depressed patients can be frustrating to family members. The frustration may lead family members to wonder whether depression is a ploy for attention or a form of manipulation. They may try to convince the depressed patient that it is all in his or her mind. Nothing could be farther from the truth.

First and foremost, depression is not something people imagine or make up. It is a horribly painful condition that causes immense suffering. Once patients recover from depression, they will often do anything to prevent it from coming back. A sixty-seven-year-old patient, who had been through both cancer and depression, once told me that if she had to have a relapse of either she'd rather it be the cancer because the depression was more horrible.

Depression is a disease felt in the mind, but it is a disease of the brain. It is as real as diabetes, high blood pressure, Parkinson's disease, and arthritis. And it needs to be taken just as seriously.

And, finally, the effects of depression are not limited to the mind. Depression affects the entire body, including the brain. As we shall see throughout this book, depression is not harmful only to mental health; it also takes an enormous toll on physical health. Older adults who fail to respect depression as a serious illness requiring treatment put their health and longevity in jeopardy.

Spending the last years of your life in a miserable state of depression and dying that way is a tragedy. Fortunately, more often than not it is an avoidable one. Treatment works, and all that is necessary is that we see depression as the serious brain disease it is rather than an expectable, normal reaction to old age. With treatment, older adults can protect their health and get their lives back, because old age is not depressing.

So here's the bottom line: Why do older adults, who have enjoyed good mental health their entire lives, become depressed for the first time in old age? It's not because old age is depressing. It's not. Depression is not a normal or inevitable part of aging. It's not a sign of weakness, all in your mind, or a condition you can handle yourself. And it's not untreatable. Older adults get depressed because the aging process causes changes in the brain's ability to handle stress and regulate emotions. In the next two chapters we'll understand this in much greater detail. Then we'll focus on the many ways depression takes a toll on health and longevity. Once we explore all this, we'll be in a good position to talk about what you can do about it.

2

WHAT CAUSES DEPRESSION?

It's Not What You Think It Is

In the last chapter, we started to look at the question "Why do older adults who have enjoyed good mental health their entire lives become depressed for the first time in old age?" I hope we completely discredited the idea that it is because old age is depressing and debunked related notions about mental health, aging, and depression. Now let's see how modern neuroscience answers the question. Older persons with no prior mental health problems get depression for the first time in old age not because old age is depressing but because depression is a brain disease to which older adults are more prone.

Before we can examine this claim, we must first define some terms. As I previously mentioned, depression is a common old-age problem. Depression is considered one of the syndromes that geriatric specialists diagnose and treat.[1] Other examples of geriatric syndromes include incontinence, frailty, immobility, falling, and dementia. Geriatric syndromes are complicated health problems that do not have a single cause. For example, infections, prostate disease, overactive bladder, limited mobility, and neurologic diseases, including dementia, can all cause urinary incontinence. Sometimes a problem may not have a single, clear-cut cause that doctors can identify. Instead multiple minor abnormalities may add up to a type of medical "perfect storm." For example, a patient with a slow gait due to Parkinson's disease or arthritis, and frequent urination due to overactive bladder or an enlarged prostate, might not become incontinent until he begins taking a water pill for high blood pressure and suddenly cannot get to the bathroom fast enough.

Heart failure is another good example. When the heart begins to give out in old age, the result is heart failure. Many diseases can cause heart failure, but the common end result is poor circulation. When the brain gives out in old age, the effects can be thought of as "brain failure." Just as circulation is the work of the heart, the mind is the work of the brain, so when the brain fails mental health problems occur. One form of "brain failure" in old age is Alzheimer's disease, and another is late-life depression.

Similar to incontinence and heart failure, depression in old age has many causes, and there are several different types. My point is that depression in the elderly is not a single disease of the brain. It is better to think of it, instead, as an end result of various possible causes that can affect brain function, alone or in conjunction.

So when we talk about depression in the elderly, we're doing a lot of lumping. At the same time, we can split geriatric depression into two types, based on the stage of life in which depression first appeared. Older adults who first developed depression when they were younger have early-onset geriatric depression. Those who get depression for the first time in old age have late-onset geriatric depression. Late-onset geriatric depression is often called late-life depression. In the United Kingdom, they call this type of depression "old-age depression," and I'll occasionally use that term too. Late-life depression is more common, because the majority of older adults with depression develop it for the first time in old age.

The distinction between early-onset depression and late-life depression is more than just timing. Early-onset geriatric depression shares many similarities with depression in younger people. Genetic makeup and the impact of present and past life hardships and setbacks are more important. In late-life depression, the aging of the brain is more important.

Before we go on, I'd like you to try to put aside your assumptions and beliefs about the mind, human behavior, mental health, and depression. Most of us base our understanding of the mind and mental health problems on our own experience. Because we are aware of our minds at work, and we feel in charge of them, we naturally believe that we know what they do and how they work. Modern brain science is gradually pulling back the curtain, allowing us a peek at the workings of the brain that make possible the amazing "wizardry" that we call the mind. In so doing, we are getting a better understanding of depression as a medical illness of the brain.

A full palette of emotions contributes to our everyday personal experience. Most of us take these emotions for granted. But have you ever wondered why we have feelings in the first place? The brain's job is to help us manage our day-to-day lives, especially our relationships with other people. Emotions help us know the importance or significance of situations and events, and what actions to take. Think about it. How could you live your life if the death of a loved one didn't make you sad or the birth of a grandchild didn't fill you with joy? Our brains are always working behind the scenes creating our inner experience, yet we are unaware of this and of how our brains work.

You can compare this to the programs on your computer. When you use a computer program—maybe you are reading an electronic version of this book on your computer—you are aware of what the computer is doing, but you are unaware of how it does it, unless you are a computer engineer. It's an oversimplification, but think of the brain as the operating system for our emotions. When your computer gets old, it may run your programs slowly or improperly. It may make mistakes, freeze, crash, or go haywire. A similar thing can happen in the aging brain.

At the risk of relying on too many electronics analogies, the brain maintains emotional equilibrium much as the onboard computer in your car handles climate control. If it gets either too hot or too cold, the system reacts to restore the temperature to the normal setting. What happens if the system goes on the fritz? That happened to me one winter. I was driving with my family in New Hampshire ski country on a bitterly cold day. The heat worked fine initially, but as it got colder an odd thing happened. The air conditioning came on, and cold air started to blow from the vents. No matter how high I turned up the heat, cold air kept coming out. The thermostat seemed to be stuck on a cold setting.

Brains manage emotions in a similar manner. All of us have periods of unpleasant feelings, such as worry, anxiety, anger, or sadness, in response to circumstances that bring on these feelings. Periods of emotional distress can last for minutes, hours, or days but ordinarily subside, to be replaced by other feelings as conditions change. Regardless of how we feel at the moment, sooner or later our mood adjusts back to normal. Not in depression.

In depression the mood "thermostat" breaks down. Instead of normal emotional reactions, patients with depression feel constantly unhappy regardless of what happens to them. They find it hard not to feel sad, gloomy, morose, pessimistic, or worried, or to experience any pleasure in life, even when happy or enjoyable things happen. It's as if their brains' emotional settings are stuck on negative feelings.

Remember Agnes, whom we met in the previous chapter? Agnes's health declined due to the effects of diabetes, congestive heart failure, and arthritis. She got physically weaker, began to fall, and was forced to move into an assisted living facility. When I met her she had severe depression. It was as if she was draped in a shroud of hopelessness and despair she couldn't shake off. Agnes's depression seemed understandable in commonsense terms. Who wouldn't be depressed, under such depressing circumstances? But this was not the whole story.

There was something more going on. The "emotional thermostat" in Agnes's brain was stuck in depression. Agnes agreed to let me treat her with antidepressant medication, and she got better. Her mood returned to normal, and her characteristically optimistic outlook was restored, even though there had been no change in her predicament. She regained her ability to make the most of it. Perhaps there was more to Agnes's depression than an understandable reaction to loss of health and independence. Obviously this comparison of brains and climate-control systems is a bit simplified. But it gives us a helpful model for seeing how depression, a mental illness, differs from normal emotional reactions.

At this point we need to pause for another definition. Have you ever thought about how you define "mental illness"? According to the Centers for Disease Control and Prevention, mental illnesses are diseases that disturb or disrupt mood, thinking, or behavior. Notice that this says nothing about the cause. Do you agree that, by this definition, Alzheimer's disease is a mental illness? I point this out because Alzheimer's disease advocates used to argue that "Alzheimer's disease is not a mental illness; it is a brain disease." This statement, meant to liberate Alzheimer's disease from the stigma of mental illness, was a well-intended public relations position. Unfortunately it reinforced the prejudice that mental illnesses such as depression are not brain diseases too.

Late-life depression is as much a brain disease as is Alzheimer's disease. Both diseases occur due to breakdown of the brain in old age. The other organs of the body show telltale signs of aging and often succumb to disease, so we shouldn't be surprised that the brain can meet a similar fate. In both depression and Alzheimer's disease, abnormal functioning of the brain causes disturbances of emotions, behavior, memory, and thinking. There are obvious and significant differences, but the most important is that Alzheimer's disease is still incurable while depression can be treated effectively.

In Alzheimer's disease, brain cells gradually die off. As more and more are lost, areas of the brain shrink and many of the mental functions the brain performs begin to fail. Early in the disease, this involves memory and language ability. As the disease worsens, the ability to recognize what objects are used for and how to use them declines. Disturbances of thinking, mood, and behavior also arise. Neuroscientists have discovered which areas of the brain are affected most in Alzheimer's disease and how this relates to its common symptoms. In similar fashion, researchers are zeroing in on the areas of the brain involved in normal emotions and depression. Many pieces of the puzzle have fallen into place, and we now have a pretty clear picture showing that depression is a brain disease.

So what actually causes the brain's emotional controls to break down? The first inkling came in the 1960s, when the monoamine hypothesis was set forth. Monoamines are important chemical messengers in the brain used to transmit signals between brain cells. They include serotonin, norepinephrine, and dopamine. This important hypothesis was based on the discovery that monoamine levels are abnormal in individuals with depression, and it proposed that these abnormal levels caused the symptoms of depression. This captured the imagination of the public, and it became commonplace to refer to depression as a chemical imbalance in the brain. Many advocates for the mentally ill and lots of depressed patients have embraced this view since it countered the stigma of depression: depression couldn't be your fault if a chemical imbalance caused it.

The monoamine hypothesis was a helpful start, and it led to treatments that have helped untold numbers of depression sufferers, but we now know that the story is much more complicated. The brain is not just a soup of chemicals in your head. It is an astonishingly complex organ made up of billions of brain cells, called neurons. Each neuron sends and receives signals to and from countless other neurons. The neurons and all their connections are organized in circuits. The circuits connect various areas of the brain in networks, which serve the various mental functions such as thinking, speaking, feeling, moving, remembering, and so forth. These networks must perform in a precisely orchestrated way for us to be healthy mentally.

You might actually think about the brain and mental health as a symphony orchestra. The sections of the orchestra—strings, woodwinds, brass, and percussion—must play in perfect harmony for the music to sound good. If just one section fouls up, noise will occur instead. Each section of the orchestra is like a network in our brains, and we are the conductors. For us to think, feel, move, and act normally, these networks must work in a carefully orchestrated way. The "noisy music" that results when one or more brain networks works improperly is mental illness. Different networks are affected in various mental illnesses including depression, anxiety, paranoia, obsessive-compulsive disorder, posttraumatic stress disorder, and Alzheimer's disease.

The evidence that disturbances in brain circuits and networks are involved in depression comes from much brain-imaging research with different types of brain scans, which provide various kinds of pictures of the brain. Computed tomography (CT) and magnetic resonance imaging (MRI) provide pictures of brain structure, and functional MRI (fMRI), single photon emission computed tomography (SPECT), and positron-emission tomography (PET) provide pictures of brain function. If the brain is a house, then CT and MRI would give pictures of the beams, plumbing, and electrical wiring, while functional MRI, SPECT, and PET show each room's temperature and where the lights are on and the water is running.

Numerous carefully conducted studies have revealed abnormalities in the brains of older persons with depression that are not present in mentally healthy elders. Key areas of the brain are smaller. These areas show chemical abnormalities and abnormally low metabolic activity.[2] White matter abnormalities are very common.[3] The white matter contains the fibers of the circuits connecting the brain's networks. The grey matter makes up the network centers. Scientists believe that these white matter abnormalities disrupt brain circuits.[4] Treatment with antidepressant medication restores the normal activity in these areas.[5] Most compelling is that some of these abnormalities revert to normal in patients who recover from depression.

Many of the white matter abnormalities seen in older adults with late-life depression represent areas of poor circulation deep inside the brain.[6] Years of high blood pressure, diabetes, elevated cholesterol, and smoking often cause this, although wear and tear over a lifetime can do it too. Other forces take their toll on the brain in various ways. As organs go, the brain is finicky. It demands more than its share of the body's energy and needs stringently controlled conditions to function properly. Chronic oxygen deprivation—from emphysema, congestive heart failure, or sleep apnea—low blood sugar, electrolyte disturbances, infections, or inflammation can have short-term or long-term effects on the brain. Years of chronic stress damage parts of the brain. Basically, when there are signs of aging-related wear and tear elsewhere in the body, it's a good bet that similar wear and tear is going on in the brain. When such wear and tear disrupts the mood-regulating circuits, depression can occur.

Many cases of late-life depression appear out of the blue, during happy times in the lives of older adults, when nothing depressing has happened. This is what we would expect from a problem that arises from disease in the brain. But other cases clearly seem triggered by depressing events. What are we to make of this?

Late-life depression is a complicated condition. The brain's job is to help individuals adjust to changing conditions, including very depressing ones, while maintaining emotional equilibrium. A brain that remains healthy in old age will continue to cope as well as it did when it was younger, maybe better. In contrast, an old brain that has been weakened by illness will be more easily overwhelmed by psychological stress. This may be truer of brains made more vulnerable to stress because of genetics or the sensitizing effects of harsh or traumatic experiences in early life.

Before we conclude this chapter, let me restate the take-home message: Mental illness, including depression, is not a normal part of aging; for most older adults, good mental health is to be expected. Depression is very common in old age but so are diabetes, high blood pressure, and arthritis. We don't consider these normal parts of aging. We treat them as diseases, and this is how we should approach depression. Few people escape sadness in old age. That's life. But old people are survivors. Those who have reached old age without ever having had depression will most likely face whatever sadness they encounter in old age without becoming depressed, as long as their brains remain fairly healthy.

Discoveries in brain science are going to force us to think differently about who we are and why we have the thoughts and feelings we do. Some will find this hard to swallow. For those with depression and other mental illnesses, it may make life easier. Gone will be the days of feeling ashamed of having depression. Stigma will be replaced with acceptance of depression as a medical illness, and older patients will receive treatment for depression as readily as they do for their high blood pressure, diabetes, and arthritis. They'll feel better, be healthier, live longer, and get their lives back.

3

DEPRESSION IN OTHER BRAIN DISEASES

Elaine was an eighty-four-year-old woman I saw in my office for depression. Her daughter, Andrea, brought her in for help, wanting her mother to have some happiness at the end of her life. I evaluated Elaine and found that she was moderately depressed. Both her parents died when Elaine was a young mother. Soon thereafter Elaine's older sister, whom she idolized, died. When Elaine was sixty, one of her sons died of a heart attack. And when she was seventy-two, her husband died. She had gone through a fairly typical period of grief and had made a good life for herself in widowhood, enjoying family, friends, and church activities. Despite the painful losses she had endured over the years, Elaine's mental health had remained good, until depression set in.

Elaine couldn't understand why she felt so depressed. She had always seen herself as someone who could cope. And there was no apparent reason for depression now: everything seemed to be going well. Her health was still fairly good. A granddaughter had just graduated from law school. Elaine had been thrilled to attend the graduation and was still bursting with pride. A grandson was getting married in a few months, to a girl Elaine really liked. She had been looking forward to the wedding. Depression now made everything seem pointless, and nothing gave her any pleasure.

Andrea was equally perplexed. Elaine had been an upbeat person who had always coped well. She assumed that something deep down had to be troubling Elaine. Maybe Elaine never really fully dealt with one or more past losses. Andrea felt certain that counseling was the solution. She thought that if a counselor could help her mother to "get it all off her chest," she would feel better and once again be the happy person Andrea had always known.

I saw Elaine and diagnosed a type of depression called major depression. We'll learn more about the different types of depression and how they are diagnosed in the next chapter. I also found something that neither Elaine nor Andrea expected: Elaine was in the earliest stage of Alzheimer's disease. Elaine had experienced some forgetfulness for a year or two, but she and Andrea had been unconcerned, thinking it was just normal aging. Unfortunately, it was more than that. As far as deep-seated, emotional troubles causing Elaine's depression, there were none in sight. Nevertheless, we began psychotherapy (what people commonly call counseling), but after three sessions, it was apparent that she didn't need it. Antidepressant medication would likely do the job alone. Elaine had been a good sport about trying psychotherapy, to ease Andrea's mind, but she was glad when I agreed that we could stop.

Through the years Elaine had been emotionally healthy and able to handle life's challenges. Her coping skills were excellent and had not let her down. Something else had caused her to get depression in old age. I suspected that the culprit was the other disease beginning to take root in her brain—Alzheimer's disease. Once Elaine's depression went away, I recommended additional treatment for Alzheimer's disease.

This was not what Andrea expected. Not only was she crestfallen by the diagnosis of Alzheimer's disease, but also she still wanted Elaine to have psychotherapy. Andrea firmly believed that people get depression "for a reason." If you do not see the reason, then you have to dig deeper, psychologically, to get it out in the open. Elaine had a different reaction. Obviously she didn't like being told she had Alzheimer's disease. But she could deal with that, as she had with other troubles in life: "You put one foot in front of the other and do the best you can," she told me. She wasn't so enthusiastic about psychotherapy. Right or wrong, she did not want to accept that she had psychological problems and needed help coping. Learning that depression is another kind of brain disease reassured her. "You mean it might be something physical, like a chemical imbalance?" she asked, with renewed self-confidence.

I meet patients and family members such as Andrea on a regular basis in my practice. In my experience, most people still think depression is a purely psychological condition, and they do not realize it has anything to do with the brain at all. I hope I convinced you in chapter 2 that depression is a disease of the brain. Just to be sure, in this chapter let's see what depression that occurs concurrently with other brain diseases further shows us about depression being a brain disease.

For centuries we have known that the mind and the brain are not separate things, despite popular views to the contrary. Nature provides us with unfortunate clues about the connection of the mind and the brain: brain damage from injury and disease causes mental symptoms. Some brain diseases, such as tumors or strokes, penetrating head wounds, and certain types of brain surgery are confined to relatively small, discrete areas of the brain. During the nineteenth and twentieth centuries, doctors caring for such patients began to observe the connection between the location of the brain damage and the pattern of mental effects it caused. This resulted in mapping the brain areas for language, short-term memory, organization and planning, arithmetic, vision, hearing, musical ability, and spatial ability. The science of understanding the relationship between the mind and the brain was thus launched. Nowadays, modern brain-scanning technologies, such as CT, MRI, fMRI, SPECT, and PET scans, which we talked about in the last chapter, allow researchers to study the same connections in healthy people and those with mental illnesses such as depression.

Older patients who become seriously ill or disabled frequently also develop depression. Heart attack, arthritis, emphysema, and chronic kidney disease are examples of diseases often associated with depression. As we will see in the chapters of part 2, the relationship between depression and such diseases is a complicated, two-way street. Brain diseases, including multiple sclerosis, stroke, traumatic brain injuries, brain tumors, epilepsy, and Alzheimer's disease, are even more complicated. Compared with disease elsewhere in the body, diseases of the brain tend to have even higher rates of depression.[1]

There are at least three reasons patients with brain diseases have depression more frequently than those with other types of disease. First, brain diseases can be the most difficult and trying of all health problems. Unlike diseases affecting other body parts, brain diseases affect speech, coordination, movement, walking, and sensation. Tremors, tics, spasms, slurred speech, disfigurement, disability, dependence, and other effects of brain diseases make life even harder for many patients. Under such circumstances, sadness, worry, embarrassment, discouragement, and anger seem natural and can evolve into depression.

The second way brain diseases bring out more depression is by directly weakening coping abilities. Coping doesn't happen by magic. It takes emotional stability, reasoning, judgment, and memory, all the mental processes that go into putting things into perspective and adapting. Diseases that disrupt the normal function of the brain can impact these abilities. In other words, emotional fortitude can be a casualty of brain disease. A person who could have found a way to adapt to cancer or a spinal cord injury might not be able to handle a stroke.

And finally, and most significantly, brain disease may damage or disrupt the brain's emotion-controlling circuits. When these circuits falter or go haywire, depression can occur.

Stroke, Alzheimer's disease, and Parkinson's disease are three brain diseases in which depression is common. The majority of the patients I treat for depression have one of these conditions. I have taken care of many of them over the years and have seen firsthand that these diseases bring on depression in all the ways I just described. For now, we'll focus on the evidence that these three brain diseases cause depression by affecting brain circuits for emotional control.

STROKE

Stroke is a sudden condition that strikes without warning. As we saw in the introduction, strokes can be life-changing catastrophes. If you have had a stroke, or know someone who has, you probably do not find it surprising that many stroke victims get depressed in its aftermath.

A stroke occurs when blood supply to part of the brain is interrupted. Either bleeding in the brain or blockage of an artery feeding an area of the brain can cause such disruption. In many ways a stroke is similar to a heart attack, and you can think of it as a "brain attack." During a stroke, the area of the brain that loses its blood supply is deprived of oxygen and essential nutrients. If this goes on long enough, the affected brain cells die.

The symptoms of a stroke reflect the loss of the functions performed by the damaged parts of the brain. Weakness, paralysis, numbness on one side of the body, and difficulty speaking are common manifestations. These occur when blood flow is cut off to motor, sensory, or language centers in the brain. Confusion, double vision, difficulty swallowing, lack of coordination, or unsteadiness are among the other possible results of a stroke. Recovery from a stroke ranges from complete to not at all and takes days, weeks, months, or longer. Many stroke victims remain permanently disabled.

Depression is very common after stroke. Forty percent of stroke patients develop depression, known as post-stroke depression, within two years.[2] Stroke victims, members of their families, and even their physicians too often consider post-stroke depression to be an understandable and expectable reaction to having a stroke. "If you'd had a stroke, wouldn't you be depressed?" illustrates the sentiment well.

No doubt having a stroke is depressing. In my experience, depressed stroke patients often feel anguish, despair, and hopelessness over their condition. But the change of attitude these patients undergo, once treatment has made the depression go away, can be dramatic: Patients whose stroke left them feeling sad, useless, worthless, guilty, and wishing to die feel happier and experience a renewed positive outlook on life. Their sense of hopelessness and uselessness gives way to a belief that they can live with their limitations, even though they might remain confined to a wheelchair or be unable to speak. Without any tangible improvement in their condition, all the psychological reasons to feel depressed persist, yet they are no longer depressed. When you see this transformation in patients, it seems pretty obvious that depression and its treatment have something to do with the workings of the brain.

Using modern brain-scanning technologies, researchers have studied thousands of stroke patients to see whether the location of the stroke in the brain matters. They discovered that, regarding depression, not all strokes are the same. In right-handed individuals, strokes on the left side of the brain more commonly lead to depression. The further forward in the brain the stroke sits, the more post-stroke depression resembles major depression, a form of severe depression affecting individuals with no other brain disease.[3] This finding led researchers to speculate that strokes cause depression by disrupting brain circuits for emotions.[4]

ALZHEIMER'S DISEASE

Older adults widely fear Alzheimer's disease, and with good reason. This dreaded condition might be the most depressing disease afflicting older adults. Alzheimer's disease causes forgetfulness, loss of memory, language problems, and gradual deterioration of all mental faculties. It robs victims of their ability to work, enjoy favorite activities, and perform day-to-day functions such as driving, banking, and cooking. In the more severe stages, patients lose the ability to dress, wash, eat, and go to the bathroom by themselves. Eventually they may fail to recognize family members or even themselves.

Does this sound depressing to you? It sure does to me. Up to half of Alzheimer's disease patients develop depression in the course of the illness, and these patients make up the largest group of the older adults I treat for depression. Some patients seek my help for depression shortly after receiving the diagnosis. The depression they have often seems to be an obvious reaction to a diagnosis of a terrible disease with a bleak future, and psychotherapy sometimes relieves such patients' depression and helps them face what lies ahead.

Surprisingly, many patients with Alzheimer's disease who get depression do not develop it until much later in the course of the disease. Somehow they cope with being diagnosed with the disease, and they learn to live with it without getting depressed. Depression strikes them much later, as the disease takes greater hold of them. No surprise there. But here's where it again gets more complicated. In some cases, depression does not set in until after patients have lost awareness of their condition. Patients in the very severe stage live in the past, no longer aware of their present condition. It is no surprise that loved ones find this stage depressing. But what explains patients' depression at this stage? It can't be a psychological reaction to a disease of which they have no awareness!

In other cases, depression makes its appearance before the telltale symptoms of Alzheimer's disease emerge. This happened to Elaine. Some older adults develop late-life depression shortly before developing Alzheimer's. As we'll see in chapter 14, a large minority of older adults with depression subsequently get Alzheimer's. Having depression increases the chance of getting Alzheimer's at a later time. In other words, sometimes depression actually "causes" Alzheimer's disease. But in other cases of depression that occurs before Alzheimer's, the Alzheimer's disease has caused the depression, but depression makes its appearance before memory impairment and other cognitive symptoms emerge. In these cases, depression is not a separate disease from Alzheimer's; it is the earliest stage. Patients with such depression do not yet recognize symptoms of Alzheimer's. If they seek help from their primary care doctors, it is because they think they have depression, not because they have noticed forgetfulness. If they see a specialist, they are more likely to go to a psychiatrist than a neurologist. Once again, these patients have no awareness they have Alzheimer's, but this time because it is too early. So they, too, have depression that cannot be explained as a psychological reaction to having Alzheimer's disease. Their depression is a symptom of the disease beginning to affect the functioning of their brains.

So how does Alzheimer's cause depression both before other symptoms appear and long after other symptoms have become severe? Alzheimer's disease is caused by the slow, accumulated death of brain cells. A process that is not yet fully understood stresses neurons to the point that they wither and die. This process probably begins in middle age but goes unnoticed for many years. As more and more brain cells die, brain circuits start to malfunction. Once this happens, the functions these circuits perform start to fail and symptoms appear.

Alzheimer's disease characteristically affects some areas of the brain earlier than others, but there is some variation from person to person. The short-term memory centers are usually the first to go, and this is why forgetfulness is generally the earliest symptom. When the frontal lobes of the brain are affected, personality change and abnormal behavior may be the first symptom. And when the emotion-regulating circuits are affected earliest, depression can be the earliest manifestation of Alzheimer's disease.[5] If, on the other hand, mood-regulating circuits are spared damage until late in the disease, then depression may not appear until the severe stage.

PARKINSON'S DISEASE

Parkinson's disease is a chronic and progressive movement disorder. Symptoms of Parkinson's include tremor, stiffness, rigidity, and slowness of movement. Those affected often have stooped posture, shuffling gait, soft or mumbling speech, poor balance, and a blank expression. Falls are common and lead to injuries.

Similar to Alzheimer's, Parkinson's is a degenerative brain disease. In this case, the death of specialized neurons that make dopamine causes the main symptoms. You may recall that dopamine is one of the monoamines. Brain circuits governing movement and other mental functions, including mood and thinking, depend on dopamine to operate normally.

Similar to stroke and Alzheimer's, Parkinson's is also an extremely difficult condition. Sufferers feel locked inside bodies that seem frozen and defy their wills. Treatment relieves some of the symptoms but is usually not fully effective. Most of the time treatment is no more than a temporary reprieve, since Parkinson's is a progressive condition without a cure. Those afflicted gradually get worse and become more and more disabled.

If this sounds bleak to you, you get the picture. As you might expect, depression affects 40 to 50 percent of patients with Parkinson's disease. Anxiety, loss of interest, and various physical complaints often go along with the depressed mood.[6] When I see one of these unfortunate patients in my practice, I always feel a strong desire to help them get better.

The depression that afflicts those with Parkinson's disease shares important similarities with depression in patients who have had a stroke or have Alzheimer's. First, it can occur either as a psychological reaction to having Parkinson's disease or directly due to brain damage caused by the disease, or both, just as it does with strokes and in Alzheimer's.[7] Second, depression also afflicts Parkinson's patients more frequently than patients with comparable degrees of physical disability from causes other than brain disease.[8]

Third, as occurs in Alzheimer's, depression in Parkinson's disease sometimes precedes the diagnostic movement symptoms. This happens when the process causing Parkinson's affects the emotion circuits earlier than the movement circuits. Mood-regulating circuits need dopamine, and Parkinson's also impacts the other brain monoamines affected in depression. In other words, it causes chemical disturbances in the brain similar to the "chemical imbalance" present in depression.

Finally, the emotion circuits affected by Parkinson's are located in the similar areas of the brain most often affected by stroke in post-stroke depression. Parkinson's patients with depression show positron-emission tomography (PET) scan abnormalities in these areas of the brain. These abnormalities are not present in Parkinson's patients who do not have depression.

And then there is the "on-off" phenomenon. This is a strange symptom that plagues some patients with Parkinson's. Patients who experience the on-off effect have dramatic fluctuations of their Parkinson's symptoms throughout the day. Their symptoms turn on and off as if controlled by a switch in the brain. It is a very curious and perplexing thing to see. One minute patients are doing fine, with few, if any, symptoms. Then suddenly their symptoms become severe: they become totally frozen and unable to move much at all, and may have trouble speaking or thinking. In many cases, the timing of the fluctuations coincides with the daily medication schedule.

The really extraordinary thing about the on-off effect is what happens when patients also have depression. During the "on" period, patients can feel perfectly happy. As soon as the "off" period starts, they are thrown into the depths of depression. Just as quickly depression goes away again when they switch back "on."[9] I can tell you that it is very striking to watch patients experience this complete and rapid change of mood. When you see this weird phenomenon, the connection between depression and brain function seems obvious: it looks as if someone is flipping a toggle switch in the brain, turning emotion circuits on and off.

CONCLUSION

We end this chapter where we began, with Elaine and Andrea. Our brief encounter with this former patient and her daughter illustrates two points. First, Elaine got depression, not because she had suffered losses, harbored some deep-down, hidden emotional problem, or just thought old age is depressing. Elaine had enjoyed robust mental health her entire life. She got depression in late life because her brain was beginning to fail as a result of Alzheimer's, a disease she did not yet know she had. Circuits in her brain were starting to malfunction, and the effect of this was depression.

Strokes and Parkinson's disease share in common with Alzheimer's the ability to cause depression by affecting the function of emotion-regulating circuits in the brain. Any health problem with detrimental effects on the brain can cause depression, and sometimes old-age wear and tear on the brain is enough to do it. The main takeaway message of this chapter is that brain diseases cause more depression than do other types of diseases because depression is itself a disease of the brain.

By now you may have realized that depression has more than one cause. In fact, depression is not a single disease; it can have different causes and there are many types. In this way depression is similar to arthritis, which is also not a single disease. There are different types of arthritis, including osteoarthritis and rheumatoid arthritis, with similar symptoms but different causes. I'd like you to keep this in mind as you begin chapter 4, which will help you recognize the different types of depression and make you aware of other conditions that mimic depression.

Our mother-daughter duo also reminds us how understanding depression as a brain disease helps some elders accept treatment. Andrea assumed that her mother's depression had a "deep-down," psychological cause. Such Freudian-style views are the rule, rather the exception, among my patients and members of their families. I suspect that this is also true of the general public. Most elders feel no shame in having Alzheimer's, Parkinson's, or a stroke, because they see these illnesses as diseases of the brain, over which they have no control. In contrast, they feel ashamed of being depressed or needing psychiatric treatment. I find that when I help my patients understand that depression is a disease of the brain, they become more receptive to treatment.

In ancient times people believed epilepsy was caused by demonic possession, and now we accept it as a disease of the brain. Depression is also a disease of the brain and a medical illness with serious consequences: it takes a toll on health and shortens life expectancy. Patients used to suffer terrible complications of diabetes, including heart disease, kidney failure, blindness, limb amputation, and premature death. As a result of widespread acceptance of treatment, most persons with diabetes can lead very normal, long lives. The same can be true of depression. Treatment of older adults with depression is effective, and it prevents tragic consequences.

4

WHAT'S IN A NAME?

Why Correct Diagnosis of Depression Matters

Nancy, a seventy-eight-year-old homemaker, had hip-replacement surgery. The operation went smoothly, but a few days later she had a heart attack, she got pneumonia, and her kidneys shut down. Things were touch and go, but Nancy pulled through . . . sort of. When Nancy finally came around she found a breathing tube in her neck and a feeding tube in her stomach. She was too weak to walk, had to use a bedpan, and was in constant pain. The doctors assured Nancy and her family that this was temporary, but she would need months of rehabilitation and possibly long-term care. A few days later, Nancy's children found her sobbing hysterically. She was gloomy, hopeless, and wanted to end it all. Nancy's children were aghast.

Do you think Nancy had depression? She certainly sounds depressed, and why wouldn't she be, considering all she was going through? Except that Nancy's diagnosis was not depression. Surprised? By the time you finish this chapter, you won't be. You'll understand why Nancy's sadness, hopelessness, and suicidal wishes do not add up to depression. And I'll bet you'll be able to tell me Nancy's correct diagnosis.

Just because someone feels sad, cries a lot, feels hopeless, or even talks about suicide does not mean he or she has depression—far from it. More goes into the diagnosis of depression, a lot more. So how do you know whether you have, or someone you care about has, depression? How does your doctor know? How is depression diagnosed?

In this chapter we're going to look at how we diagnose depression in older adults. First we'll describe the symptoms of depression in detail. Then we'll see how a number of conditions masquerade as depression. After that we will go through the diagnoses of different types of depression and why correct diagnosis matters. Finally, we will see how depression can look different in the very old and how this often muddles the picture.

If you find all this confusing, that's okay. If you take away an understanding that there is more than meets the eye in diagnosing depression, and get a feel for what depression is and what it is not, then you'll be able to work with your doctors to receive the right diagnosis and treatment.

DIAGNOSIS MATTERS

Did you know that "depression" is not a diagnosis at all but only a symptom of a problem that has many possible diagnoses? Don't feel bad if you answered no. Most people, including the majority of healthcare professionals, see depression as a single condition, present whenever anyone is excessively sad, blue, or down for any period of time. Depression is far more complicated. It is a group of mood disorders, all sharing common symptoms including unhappiness, sadness, emptiness, irritability, and negative or pessimistic thinking.[1]

Actually, it's the same way with many common physical illnesses. Take low back pain, a common problem among older adults. Like depression, low back pain is a symptom, not a diagnosis. Some common causes of low back pain in older adults are osteoarthritis, spinal stenosis, "slipped disk," and compression fracture. Each one of these diagnoses requires a somewhat different treatment, so knowing which one is correct makes a difference. Depression is no different.

If you have low back pain, your doctor can examine you and run tests to determine the cause and make the correct diagnosis. It's no different in psychiatry, except there are very few tests in psychiatry. Cutting-edge brain scans, such as positron-emission tomography (PET) and functional MRI (fMRI), have opened a window into the brain through which researchers can "see" depression. But in routine clinical practice all of the diagnoses of depression are still defined by their symptoms. Sad mood, crying, and even talk about suicide are among the core symptoms of depression. But they are symptoms of some other things, too, as we shall see.

Exact diagnosis is just as critical in depression as it is for any other medical problem. Having the correct diagnosis ensures that those who need treatment get the right type. And it spares others from treatment they do not need at all. Accurate diagnosis can make the difference between cure and calamity.

A BIT OF "BIBLE" THUMPING

Because depression is diagnosed based on symptoms, let's talk about how mental health professionals do this. The *Diagnostic and Statistical Manual of Mental Disorders*, fifth edition (*DSM-5*) is the bible of psychiatric diagnosis. It is a catalog of diagnoses and the criteria—lists of symptoms—that should be used to make each diagnosis. It is used worldwide for diagnosing depression and other mental health problems.

Major depressive disorder is one *DSM-5* diagnosis. It is a particularly severe form of depression and an important one. When psychiatrists talk about depression, it is usually shorthand for major depressive disorder. If they mean another *DSM-5* diagnosis, you can often tell, even if they have not spelled it out.

When non–mental health specialists refer to depression, they do so in a one-size-fits-all way, treating depression as a diagnosis and not just a symptom that has to be diagnosed. Some may not even be aware that there are different diagnoses for depression. This results in fuzzy diagnoses, which can lead to treatment errors. Being specific matters. You may want to ask your doctor what type of depression he or she thinks you have.

Think about the last time you had a headache. You probably took an over-the-counter pain reliever and it went away. But what if it didn't after a few weeks? You would go to your doctor expecting more than a confirmation of what you already know, "yes, you have a headache," followed by a prescription for a stronger painkiller. You would want a careful evaluation to find out whether you have a tension headache, a sinus headache, or a migraine headache, because each of these has a different treatment. You might also hope that your doctor would order tests to rule out a brain tumor. In other words, you would expect a more specific diagnosis than "headache." Once again, depression is no different.

When I see an older adult who might have some form of depression, I usually try to find out how many of the symptoms of major depressive disorder he or she has. This helps me know whether the problem is depression at all or one of the masqueraders we'll get to soon. Once I'm satisfied that some form of depression is present, I try to decide whether it is major depressive disorder or another depressive disorder. I use the symptoms of major depression as a guidepost, so let's go through them carefully.

- Course: Major depression is a condition that is present, on most days, for at least two weeks but usually much longer. It can go on for months or years and may become chronic.
- Mood: Usually sad, gloomy, hopeless, irritable, or empty. Older patients may say they feel down in the dumps, nervous, easily upset, or blah.
- Thinking: Patients complain about difficulty thinking or concentrating. They often have trouble making decisions, even trivial ones. For example, choosing what clothes to wear for the day may feel overwhelming.
- Thoughts: A tendency to dwell on worries or negative thoughts is common. The worries are often blown out of proportion. Patients may feel worthless, useless, or unjustifiably guilty. Older adults often feel they have become a burden to their families, who would be better off without them. Belief that all efforts are futile, including medical care, may be present. Thoughts about death may include wishes to die or ideas about suicide, including plans for carrying it out.
- Behavior: Patients may be jumpy, fidgety, tense, or restless, with pacing, handwringing, or rubbing, scratching, or picking the skin. They may be upset, overwhelmed, or frustrated by minor problems. Sometimes sluggishness, slow movements, and delayed, slow, or soft, mumbling speech occur instead. Patients may with-

draw in bed, or sit in a dark room, saying little. Self-neglect is common, often leading to serious health problems.

- Cognition: Depressed patients are often forgetful and inattentive. They may seem "out of it." Cognitive symptoms may be severe enough to mimic Alzheimer's disease.

- Neurovegetative symptoms: No, carrots and broccoli don't get depression. This odd word, "neurovegetative," refers to bodily functions having to do with physical needs and desires, such as eating, sleeping, and sexual activity. Depressed patients have low energy and little or no motivation and interest in activities. There may be loss of sex drive. Patients lose the ability feel pleasure or enjoy life. Decreased appetite and weight loss are common. In some forms of major depression, appetite is increased and there may be weight gain. Patients with depression usually have trouble sleeping. Insomnia can occur during any part of the night, but the tendency to wake up in the early morning hours and not be able to fall back to sleep is particularly diagnostic. Increased sleep can occur in some cases.

- Physical symptoms: While depression is primarily a disturbance of mood, physical symptoms are also common. Aches and pains may appear or get worse. Vision or hearing problems may worsen. Other symptoms can include bowel or bladder complaints, difficulty breathing, chest pain, and feeling dizzy or off balance. Because older adults can have physical symptoms for so many reasons, their presence in depression makes depression easy to overlook.

- Severity: Major depressive disorder causes clinically significant distress or impairment of day-to-day functioning, or both.

I memorized the symptoms of major depression a long time ago, but I don't expect you to. I just want you to have a feeling for what major depressive disorder and similar forms of serious depression are like. Throughout this book, whenever we talk about the types of depression that can impact health and longevity, we'll be talking about major depressive disorder or conditions similar to it.

Here is where diagnosing depression starts to get confusing. Older adults with depression can have other symptoms not on the list. And as we will see in the next section, other conditions can mimic depression.

So try to keep the list of symptoms of major depressive disorder in mind, because we will use it as a frame of reference as we talk about different diagnoses of depression and other conditions that can be mistaken for depression.

CONDITIONS THAT MASQUERADE AS DEPRESSION

Before you accept any treatment for depression, make sure you really have it. A number of conditions masquerade as depression. It's especially easy to be fooled if you have had depression before, as happened to Kevin.

Kevin was a seventy-nine-year-old retired high school mathematics teacher. He'd always been energetic and enthusiastic, and had stayed active in retirement.

Two years earlier I had treated him for depression. Kevin's depression left him emotionally empty. He was sluggish and had no interest in doing anything; he felt down on himself, useless, and worthless. Three psychotherapy sessions and treatment with an antidepressant medication was all it took for Kevin to get better. After three months and a total of six visits, Kevin felt back to normal. I saw Kevin for regular checkups for two years and then discharged him.

Eighteen months later Kevin came back to see me. For three months he'd been feeling tired and sluggish, and his usual energy had vanished. Kevin went to see his primary care physician. But a physical examination revealed nothing conclusive. Kevin's primary care physician "reassured" him that he was just slowing down due to old age.

Things got worse. Kevin lost his motivation to do anything. He mostly lay on the couch watching television and feeling sorry for himself. Kevin's wife, Betty, realized he might be depressed again. He had all the same symptoms as before. She brought Kevin to see me.

When I saw Kevin he was very discouraged and frustrated, but he didn't have depression. Sure, his mood was low; his energy, poor; and his motivation to do things, nonexistent. But something didn't fit. In the two months between seeing his primary care physician and coming to see me, Kevin had developed swelling of his feet and ankles, and climbing a flight of stairs left him winded. I listened to his lungs and heard congestion. Rather than conclude Kevin had depression, I referred him back to his primary care physician for a closer look. This time, he found that Kevin was in congestive heart failure. In hindsight, this had been brewing all along, but the usual signs were not yet detectable when Kevin first saw his primary care doctor. Kevin's primary care physician treated Kevin for congestive heart failure. This got Kevin back on track. His usual energy, enthusiasm, and motivation returned, and he resumed most of his activities. Lo and behold, Kevin didn't have a relapse of depression.

Low energy, lack of interest, sluggishness, loss of appetite, poor sleep, and aches and pains are symptoms not only of depression. They occur as part of many other medical conditions affecting older adults as well. The telltale diagnostic symptoms may not be present early on in illnesses such as congestive heart failure, thyroid disease, chronic kidney disease, or diabetes. As you might imagine, feeling crummy without knowing why can be discouraging and depressing. I think you can see how easy it might be to mistake this for depression.

As Kevin's situation shows, misattributing another condition to depression can result in a delay in diagnosing and treating serious conditions such as congestive heart failure. Being savvy about this possibility allows you to ask your doctors questions to ensure this doesn't happen to you or someone you care about. Let's go through some particular conditions that can easily be mistaken for depression.

Apathy

Apathy is a condition characterized by loss of interest, low motivation and ambition, and poor initiative. Patients with apathy are not usually down, sad, or negative, and they do not have the guilt, hopelessness, despair, or thoughts of death experienced by those with depression. Apathetic individuals seem indifferent and are content doing nothing. Family members often refer to them as "lumps on a log." Because of this, apathy is often mistaken for depression.

Apathy is common in Parkinson's disease, stroke, Lewy body dementia, progressive supranuclear palsy, normal pressure hydrocephalus, frontotemporal dementia, traumatic brain injury, hypothyroidism, cardiovascular disease, and Alzheimer's disease.

It is important to make sure that apathy is not incorrectly diagnosed as depression. Treatments for depression will most likely not help apathy. Worse yet, the selective serotonin reuptake inhibitor (SSRI) antidepressants sometimes make apathy worse.

SLEEP APNEA

Patients with sleep apnea seek medical help because of severe daytime sleepiness. Such patients are often puzzled by their symptoms. They sleep soundly all night and can't understand why they feel so sleepy during the day. Their spouses often recognize the problem because the characteristic heavy snoring keeps them up at night. Being awake, they happen to notice that the person frequently stops breathing, gasps for air, or awakens startled.

Younger patients with sleep apnea go to their doctor because the daytime tiredness makes them fall asleep at work, which does little for their job security. Sleep apnea is more likely to go undetected among the elderly. One reason is that older retirees don't have bosses to satisfy. Not having a job, or many other places to go to, they are free to nap all day. Some assume that tiredness is a normal part of aging. It's not. And if these individuals already have mild dementia, they may not think to mention their tiredness to family members or their doctor.

Feeling too tired, elders with sleep apnea may beg off activities or outings, claiming they are not interested. Family members who find them in bed all the time may assume the cause is depression.

Here again, correct diagnosis matters. Antidepressant medications do no good in sleep apnea. Some can make sleep apnea worse. Even more worrisome is that left untreated sleep apnea increases the risk of high blood pressure, stroke, heart attack, and dementia—all avoidable fates! Proper diagnosis and treatment of sleep apnea may require consultation with a sleep specialist and overnight sleep studies.

Dementia

You may recall from chapter 3 that the relationship between depression and dementia is complicated. Maybe you still have a headache from thinking about it. Sorry, but it is even more confusing. Not only does depression sometimes occur as the first symptom of dementia, symptoms of dementia are also easily mistaken for depression.

Catherine the Librarian

Catherine was a seventy-four-year-old high school librarian who retired on her seventieth birthday. The death of her husband, ten years earlier, had been hard, but she continued to find meaning in her work. Playing a part in the education of class after class made her feel vital. Retirement had been another difficult adjustment, but she found new ways to stay active and remained well emotionally.

Six months before I met Catherine, her primary care physician had prescribed a low dose of an antidepressant for depression. When she did not improve, Catherine's doctor referred her to me for advice about a more effective treatment. I evaluated Catherine and discovered that her problem wasn't depression at all. It was dementia.

Catherine's children, who lived nearby, had noticed a change in her behavior. She stopped going out to community activities and made excuses to avoid outings with friends. She claimed these things no longer interested her. Catherine also seemed helpless, which was a startling departure from her can-do personality. She stayed home and began spending more and more time in bed. And she became lax and indifferent about paying bills, doing laundry, and buying fresh groceries. She passively allowed her children to take over. They were happy to help but also deeply worried. They knew something was wrong and guessed that she must be depressed.

Her daughter Beverly arranged an appointment with Catherine's primary care physician. When Catherine's doctor heard the story, she agreed that it sounded like depression, and she prescribed an antidepressant. Here's the problem. While such a change in behavior often signifies depression, in Catherine's case it was really due to dementia.

Catherine was a bright, intelligent person who had gone to a prestigious college and then on for a master's degree. She had been highly capable and easily juggled working, managing the household, and volunteering for the local historical society. Dementia crept in undetected. Catherine forgot how to do things. She didn't realize what was wrong; she only knew she felt insecure and unsure of herself, an unfamiliar and worrisome feeling. A sense of foreboding about going out set in. Catherine worried she might get lost or run into friends or acquaintances whose names she might not recall. It was easier to ignore bills than deal with not remembering how to write a check. Not knowing what to do, she convinced herself that, at her age, napping was a good idea. Staying in bed was safe, and she did this more and more. Withdrawing to bed is something persons with depression do to avoid a world that feels too overwhelming, but those with dementia sometimes do the same thing to avoid facing a world that has become too confusing.

Involuntary Emotional Control Disorder

Patients with this condition have sudden bouts of crying, often out of the blue. Others suffer from attacks of laughter. The actual medical term for this condition is pseudobulbar affect, PBA for short. PBA is a disorder of emotional control. Laughing is pleasant, and even good for you, but can be enormously troublesome: bursting out with hysterical laughter during a church sermon or funeral does not make you popular. You can think of PBA as emotional incontinence—embarrassing, inconvenient, and messy.

Old age can be a difficult and trying time of life. When an older adult who has had sad things happen frequently breaks out crying, it's common sense to conclude they have depression, unless you know about, and suspect, PBA. This is especially likely to happen when the crying spells are triggered by something emotional. Alvin illustrates this pretty clearly.

Alvin's Story

Alvin saw combat during the Korean conflict. He had been through grisly, terrifying hand-to-hand combat yet survived, unscathed physically or emotionally. Recently Alvin had started to cry a lot. Mostly this appeared out of the blue. But other times, war movies, which had never bothered him, brought it out. Alvin's son concluded that his dad had bottled up war-related depression that was finally coming out. This was a very plausible explanation, except that Alvin was not depressed. Alvin was pretty emphatic that watching war movies did not make him feel sad or upset. And he had no other symptoms of depression. Alvin had PBA.

During the prior year, Alvin had fallen four times. Each time he hit his head. Cumulative minor traumatic brain injuries gave Alvin PBA.

The really odd thing about PBA is that the emotional outbursts do not reflect the person's inner feelings. This is because PBA is a disturbance of emotional expression, not mood. Patients often comment, "I'm crying like a baby, but I don't feel sad," a very strange and disturbing feeling. A few of my patients with PBA admitted they were afraid they were going "really crazy." Once I explained PBA to them, they were quite relieved. Knowing where the problem came from, some of these patients decided just to live with it rather than have treatment.

Aprosodia

In a way, aprosodia is the opposite of PBA. Aprosodia is a condition of dulled or absent emotional expression. In right-handed individuals, damage to the right side of the brain can cause aprosodia.

Patients with aprosodia speak in a monotone and have little facial expression. This gives the impression that they are emotionally withdrawn, indifferent, or empty. Others commonly take this to be an indication of depression. Strokes are a typical cause of aprosodia. In my experience, patients with aprosodia are commonly misdiagnosed with depression.

Once again, similar to PBA, there is a disconnection between outward expression of emotions and inner feelings. Patients with aprosodia do not feel depressed, and they do not benefit from treatment for depression. Once they and their family members understand what is going on, everyone feels more comfortable.

Delirium

If you've ever known someone who was seriously ill in the hospital and seemed really out of it, he or she probably had delirium. Delirium occurs when serious illness or surgery makes the brain go haywire. Pneumonia, dehydration, electrolyte imbalances, out-of-control diabetes, stroke, and narcotic pain medications are frequent causes of delirium. Delirium is very common among older hospital patients and nursing home residents.

Delirium has many symptoms and is thus easily mistaken for other psychiatric conditions. The foremost manifestation of delirium is clouded, foggy thinking with reduced awareness of the environment and difficulty paying attention. Delirious patients may seem dazed and unaware of their surroundings or be excessively vigilant, reacting with fear to mundane background events that people ordinarily ignore. Sleep is erratic. The symptoms come and go, and patients may have calm periods, during which they seem lucid. Other symptoms include confused thinking, disorientation, mood swings, paranoid fears and other irrational beliefs, and hallucinations. Cognitive impairment is common and often includes disorientation and short-term memory impairment. Mood swings may occur, and periods of sadness, crying, or talking about death may lead to incorrect diagnosis of, and treatment for, depression.

I hope you never experience delirium, but if you have, and you're reading this book, you have probably recovered fully. With proper medical attention, delirium clears up. But it has to be recognized for what it is. Often it is mistaken for—you guessed it—depression.

How does this mistake happen? Confusion, disorientation, bewilderment, and inattention can fly under the radar of doctors and nurses alike. Not until the patient starts to cry and talks about wanting to die does anyone take notice. It's natural to conclude that such a person has depression because of the awful illness they are dealing with. By the way, have you figured out that Nancy, the woman I described at the start of this chapter, had delirium?

Misdiagnosing delirium as depression can be catastrophic. Giving a delirious person antidepressant medications may make the delirium worse. And causes of delirium are often life threatening, so any delay in diagnosis can be dire.

Failure to Thrive

Failure to thrive, FTT for short, in the elderly is not a single disease or even a unique medical condition. It is a state of decline characterized by weight loss, poor appetite, and malnutrition. Patients with FTT dwindle away. They become inactive, weak or infirm, prone to dehydration and infections, and susceptible to injury. They may appear mentally dull, sluggish, feeble, or depressed. In fact, depression can be one cause of failure to thrive.

But depression is not the only or even main cause of failure to thrive. Congestive heart failure, chronic lung disease, or chronic kidney disease are often culprits. Alcohol abuse, swallowing problems, and factors interfering with grocery shopping and cooking, such as social isolation, immobility, poor vision, or dementia, may bring it about. Often there is not a single cause but several factors acting together. I think you can see how easy it might be to see FTT as depression, even when there is no depression present.

DEPRESSION OR DEPRESSIONS?

When individuals have depression, psychiatrists usually try to determine which symptoms of major depressive disorder they have. If their symptoms fit the pattern, then that will probably be the diagnosis. If not, they look for an alternative diagnosis that fits the picture better. So let's go through the diagnoses of depression and see how each differs from major depressive disorder.

Major Depressive Disorder

Mental health specialists focus on major depressive disorder for a few reasons. It stands out clearly as a disease, being identifiable in distinct episodes of illness. It is severe and disabling. And it is common and recurring. We went through the symptoms already, so I won't repeat them now.

Psychotic Depression

One particularly severe type of depression is psychotic depression, officially called major depression with psychotic features. An easier way to think of it, however, is depression with irrational thoughts. This is a very severe form of depression, as you will now see.

Fred was a retired financial advisor who had enjoyed good mental health. At the age of seventy-two, Fred became severely depressed. He began to feel guilty that he had made terrible investment decisions as a young man. He then started to believe that these decades-old investment decisions caused the current world financial crisis. He sat mumbling over and over, "It's all my fault." His family tried to reason with him, but it did no good. Fred felt terrified that officials from the World Bank were going to seek his extradition for trial before the United Nations Security Council. He decided that the only way to spare his family public disgrace would be to commit suicide. Fortunately, before

Fred did anything harmful, he was hospitalized and treated for depression.

Psychosis means being out of touch with reality. In psychotic depression, the nature of the delusions and hallucinations usually reflects the depressed feelings, as Fred's did. Often there is a firm belief that a situation is hopeless, even when problems are only mild and easily solved. Older adults may refuse needed medical treatment, believing they either deserve to be punished or are beyond help.

Often psychotic symptoms go unrecognized. While the emotional manifestations of depression are apparent to others, older adults commonly keep their irrational thoughts to themselves and may not disclose these symptoms to their family members or doctors. Thus it may take some time, even for geriatric psychiatrists, to detect psychosis and diagnose psychotic depression.

Patients with psychotic depression must take both an antipsychotic medication and an antidepressant. Antidepressants alone rarely work. One reason older adults with depression do not get better is that psychotic depression has not been recognized and antipsychotic medication has not been prescribed.

Persistent Depressive Disorder (Dysthymia)

Dysthymia is very similar to major depressive disorder. The symptoms of dysthymia and major depressive disorder are identical. The conditions differ only in severity and duration. Dysthymia is milder. Patients have fewer symptoms than with major depression. But dysthymia is a longer-lasting condition. It must be present at least two years before it can be diagnosed. You may recall that major depression can be diagnosed after just two weeks.

If major depressive disorder is a raging forest fire, dysthymia is a smoldering one. It is easier for people to live with dysthymia, so they are less likely to get help. In some ways this makes it more detrimental to health. Once a forest fire is extinguished, the forest can grow back. With a constantly smoldering forest fire, there is no chance for this.

Substance/Medication-Induced Depressive Disorder

Whenever any type of depression is triggered by use of prescription medications, illicit drugs, or alcohol, this is the diagnosis. The blood pressure medications hydralazine, reserpine, and alpha-methyldopa are strongly linked to depression. Beta-blockers also have been implicated in depression, but the evidence against them is not as solid. Alcohol, narcotics, sedatives, and other drugs of abuse are often associated with depression. Even medications prescribed by thoughtful and caring physicians can cause problems.

Depressive Disorder Due to Another Medical Condition

Depressive disorder due to another medical condition is just what it says: depression caused by another illness. Post-stroke depression is a clear-cut example. In the last chapter we saw that Alzheimer's and Parkinson's also cause depression. Traumatic brain injury, multiple sclerosis, hypothyroidism, Cushing's syndrome, and deficiencies of vitamins B_{12}, D, and folic acid are other examples of diseases that can cause or contribute to depression.

Bipolar Depression

Some episodes of depression are caused by bipolar disorder. Older adults may know this as manic-depressive illness, an older name for this complicated mood disorder. Bipolar disorder causes a form of depression called bipolar depression.

Bipolar disorder usually starts in the adolescent or young-adult years. Some cases begin in old age, but most likely this is a different animal entirely, caused by brain injury, stroke, or dementia. Throughout the lives of patients with bipolar disorder, episodes of depression and mania come and go, usually at different times. Between episodes, some patients are well and lead perfectly normal lives, but many don't shake the symptoms completely, which can be chronic and disabling.

Episodes of bipolar depression are similar to those of major depressive disorder, with some exceptions. Patients with bipolar depression tend to sleep and eat more. You may recall that insomnia and poor appetite are the rule in major depressive disorder.

Manic episodes are the opposite of depression. When manic, patients are elated, silly, high, or angry. They have a puffed-up, inflated sense of themselves and have highfalutin, grandiose ideas. These can be psychotic. For example, one of my patients thought God revealed the secret of world peace to him, and he drove to Washington, D.C., to tell the president, who he was sure would welcome him into the Oval Office. The Secret Service wasn't very hospitable. During manic episodes, patients have increased energy and reduced need for sleep. Patients may become hyperactive and take on various, sometimes bizarre, projects. Risky behavior, with poor judgment and indiscretion, is common, possibly leading to harmful consequences. To qualify for the diagnosis, a manic episode must last at least one week.

Bipolar depression is often severe; and the need for treatment, urgent and compelling. Doctors often prescribe antidepressant medications, sometimes without realizing the patient has bipolar disorder. This can cause serious trouble. Patients with bipolar depression who receive antidepressant medication often improve quickly. But when given to a person with bipolar depression, antidepressant medications can trigger a switch from depression to mania, and mania can be riskier and more destructive than depression. I once had a patient who gambled away his entire fortune, nearly three million dollars, after his primary care doctor gave him antidepressants and he became manic. Ouch! And use of antidepressants may cause bipolar disorder to get worse, with more frequent episodes that are harder to treat.

Adjustment Disorder with Depression

Adjustment disorder with depression is a period of depression triggered by a clear emotional stress, such as retirement or moving. The depression is not severe enough for a diagnosis of major depressive disorder, but it is more severe than would normally be expected under the circumstances. So normal grief is not considered an adjustment disorder. Timing is important. The symptoms must start within three months of the stress and last no more than six months.

Correct diagnosis of this condition matters because adjustment disorders often go away by themselves. Many patients do not need treatment. Reassurance that they are not seriously mentally ill and will get better on their own is often enough. Some cases are severe enough that treatment with antidepressant medication or psychotherapy may be appropriate.

Bereavement Depression

One of the sad challenges of getting older is grief. The longer you live, the more deaths of loved ones you bear. Grief is a part of life that is depressing. But where does normal grief end and depression begin?

Serious depression that is more than normal grief is sometimes called bereavement depression. Being able to distinguish one from the other helps avoid two possible errors. The first is ignoring serious depression because we think sadness and grief are just normal parts of aging. The second is turning normal grief into a medical illness and giving older adults antidepressant medications they do not need.

Normal grief is necessary and healthy—painful but healthy. Grief helps the bereaved, regardless of age, cope with their loss in a psychologically sound way. In my experience, too often older adults are not given the chance to experience mourning. They are too readily given antidepressant medications, in the absence of diagnosed bereavement depression.

So how can you tell the difference between normal grief and bereavement depression? In grief, depressive feelings come and go. Feelings of despair, longing, and self-pity are usually mixed in with loving memories of the deceased. The person in mourning can be distracted from their grief, at least temporarily, and they may cheer up briefly. In contrast, in depression, low mood and negative thinking are fairly constant and impossible to shake off. Grief does not usually impact the mourner's self-esteem, whereas older adults with bereavement depression may feel worthless.

Guilty feelings may trouble both healthy mourners and those with bereavement depression. The difference in the guilt can be subtle. In normal grief, the mourner may feel guilty about something bearing on the death. For instance, the mourner might think *if only I had called the doctor sooner* or *I should have tried harder to get him (or her) to quit smoking*. In contrast, in depression the guilt may be more self-berating: *if I had just been a better wife*. Or it may seem more irrational: *if only I had not insisted on taking that job in Minneapolis after the baby was born (fifty years ago)*. In normal grief, mourners can see that their guilt is unjustified, but in depression mourners may be impervious to reason. Finally, suicidal thoughts can be seen in depression but are much less likely in normal grief.

Severity and duration are two additional differences. Grief usually lasts three to six months. Therefore, it is best to avoid treatment prior to three months if possible, unless symptoms are severe.[2] When bereaved older adults do not function well, eat poorly, or neglect their personal hygiene and health care, treatment is needed right away. Even when grief symptoms are not this severe, if the period of grief seems abnormally prolonged, treatment may be a good idea.

Bereavement depression is not an official diagnosis but a term geriatric psychiatrists use. Most cases of bereavement depression will be diagnosed as major depressive disorder.

Seasonal Affective Disorder

Known as SAD for short, seasonal affective disorder is a depressive illness that returns annually. Persons with SAD usually notice their symptoms starting to return in the late fall, and by late winter they start to feel better again.

SAD is another one of those diagnoses that is not recognized in *DSM-5*. The closest fit is usually major depressive disorder. *DSM-5* recognizes this pattern of depression with the designation "with seasonal pattern." So even though the public recognizes SAD, and psychiatrists and other healthcare professionals use the term, if you have SAD you might be diagnosed as having major depression disorder with seasonal pattern. To qualify for this diagnosis, you must have had at least two annual episodes of SAD.

SAD is easily confused with winter blues and holiday blues. According to the National Institutes of Health, winter blues is a milder form of SAD that does not affect daily functioning and clears up by itself.[3] SAD also eventually goes away but is usually too severe to ride out until spring. Holiday blues refers to the melancholic doldrums that strike some people during the Christmas season. Holiday blues is a mild condition that goes away on its own.

It is a mistake to equate SAD with the winter blues or holiday blues. SAD is a serious form of depressive illness. It is a brain disease triggered by the effect shorter winter days, with less sunlight, have on the twenty-four-hour biological clock of those vulnerable to this condition.

OLD PEOPLE DO NOT READ THE *DSM-5*

Now I have not done a survey, nor have I bothered to find out whether anyone else has, but I'll bet that not too many older adults have read the *DSM-5*. That's not to say they couldn't, or shouldn't. My guess is that they have much better things to do with their time. Good for them. But it poses an added challenge in diagnosis for everyone else. You see, not being up on *DSM-5*, older adults with depression do not know what symptoms they are supposed to have, so they often have symptoms that do not clearly fit any diagnosis. Yes, you are absolutely right. I am being flippant. But you'll appreciate why in a minute.

One diagnostic challenge in geriatrics is that diseases of all kinds can look very different in older adults compared with younger people. The usual criteria we use to diagnose illness may not apply as well to older adults. Take a heart attack, for example. The classic symptoms doctors look for to recognize heart attacks include crushing chest pain that radiates down the left arm and into the neck and jaw, nausea, vomiting, shortness of breath, and sweating. But many older patients do not have these symptoms during a heart attack. Their only symptoms may be feeling miserable, sluggish, fatigued, tired, or subdued. They may stay in bed, thinking they have the flu, and only discover they had a heart attack at some later time when it shows up on a routine cardiogram. Late-life depression does not always look the way we expect it to either.

So was it a waste of time to go over the *DSM-5* diagnoses of depression? Absolutely not. Much late-life depression looks similar enough to depression in younger persons, just a little grayer, so to speak. The symptom patterns for each condition are still good diagnostic guideposts. We just have to allow for the effects of aging.

One important difference is that neurovegetative symptoms are less helpful as clues to the presence of severe depression in older adults than in younger people. The reason is that lack of energy, poor appetite, insomnia, and loss of sexual drive are also symptoms of so many other diseases affecting older adults, including congestive heart failure, emphysema, and arthritis. Because these symptoms are so widespread, they are not good diagnostic hints. Doctors ignore depression as a possible cause.

Another challenge in geriatrics is the occurrence of depression without sadness.[4] I know, this sounds counterintuitive. But some older adults actually have depression without feeling down. They think depressing thoughts without having a depressed mood. They may think they are worthless and useless, view their situation as hopeless, wish to die, and have suicidal thoughts but do not feel sad, blue, down in the dumps, or gloomy. Older patients with depression without sadness may be nervous and tense instead, and be diagnosed with anxiety and treated with antianxiety medications. Some patients say they have no feelings at all, while still others are angry and irritable.[5] I have seen many cases of older adults who became uncharacteristically short tempered and were put on tranquilizers by their primary care physicians, who did not recognize that depression was the problem.

And finally there is the depression-executive dysfunction syndrome, a presentation of late-life depression that I see often in my practice.[6] In this type of depression, executive dysfunction accompanies many of the usual depressive symptoms. Executive dysfunction refers to a breakdown of the command and control faculties of the brain that enable us to manage our lives. The executive functions include focusing, planning, organizing, setting goals, getting started and knowing when to stop, and being flexible.

People with impaired executive functions usually seem disorganized. They can be distractible and have trouble focusing on and completing tasks. Difficulty getting started on jobs gives the appearance of laziness, apathy, or a lack of motivation. Once they get under way, they have a hard time shifting gears to do something else. They keep repeating the same action long after it is obvious they should stop. This makes them seem rigid, inflexible, or stubborn. You can imagine that older adults with both depressive symptoms and executive dysfunction can be severely disabled, and this might baffle and frustrate their family members.

Let's try to put all this into a practical perspective you can use. Think of *DSM-5* diagnoses of depression as round holes and older patients with depression as square pegs that belong in those round holes. Now, I certainly do not mean to imply that my patients or other older adults with depression are "squares." Far from it. Some of them are pretty cool, once they recover from their depression. It's just that if we only diagnose depression when older adults fit into a *DSM-5* "round hole," we will fail to diagnose the disorder in many older adults who have it. Family members, eldercare workers, primary care physicians, and other specialists often identify depression correctly. If you fit nicely in a round hole, you can feel more confident that some form of treatment of depression might be right for you. On the other hand, if you seem to be a square peg, don't jump to conclusions. Be aware of the different possibilities we covered in this chapter, ask questions, and seek help from a geriatric psychiatry specialist with the expertise to recognize the unusual ways depression can appear in older adults.

CONCLUSION

I hope that I have not totally confused you or given you the impression that diagnosing geriatric depression is a hopeless mess. It is not really that bad, but it does help if you have a lot of experience, know what to look for, and are at least a little flexible in seeing when square pegs fit good enough in round holes.

I wrote this book to alert you about the unseen dangers of depression. In the chapters of part 2, you will see how depression can worsen your health, make you old before your time, and shorten your life. Warnings do little good unless there is something you can do about it. So in part 3 I'm going to tell you what you need to know to beat depression to stay healthier and live longer. For now, let's finish this chapter with some strategies you can use to help get the right diagnosis of depression.

- Keep in mind that lists of symptoms, including those you might read in the *DSM-5*, are not by themselves enough to properly diagnose mental health problems. It takes professional training, experience, and judgment.
- Remember that the accepted descriptions and the lists of symptoms of a disease may not apply to all older adults. Diseases of all kinds look different in older adults.
- Avoid jumping to the conclusion that older persons who cry, seem down in the dumps, or talk about suicide necessarily have depres-

sion. Having reasons to be depressed does not mean you have depression. Not everything that looks like depression is depression.

- Don't forget that many other conditions masquerade as late-life depression. Always be on the lookout for delirium in hospitalized persons and among residents of long-term care facilities or those who have been sick, especially if there have been a number of medication changes. And before accepting that depression is the correct diagnosis, make sure a thorough medical evaluation has been done.

- Look at the course of the problem over time. Depression that warrants professional attention is usually present constantly, over extended periods of time. Serious depression really seems to take hold of the person and doesn't let go. People with depression seem unable to shake off the condition.

- Don't be satisfied with "depression" for a diagnosis. Ask your healthcare provider for a specific diagnosis. If he or she seems perplexed by your request, clarify that you mean the *DSM-5* diagnosis. This is your chance to see how well your healthcare professional understands depression and, in so doing, hopefully nudge the quality of treatment up a notch.

Part II

Depression Is Bad for You: How Depression Can Wreck Your Health and Shorten Your Life

5

"WHAT YOU DON'T KNOW WON'T HURT YOU"

Wrong! The More You Know about Depression, the Healthier You Can Be

In our desire to stay healthy and prevent disease, we are pretty good about paying attention to blood pressure, cholesterol, weight (well, maybe not so much), smoking, diabetes, and heart rhythm problems, such as atrial fibrillation. We get colonoscopies, mammograms, blood tests, and prostate exams. And we try to eat right, exercise, and drink in moderation, again maybe not so much, but at least we know we should. Yet we pay little or no attention to depression.

Few people appreciate the toll untreated depression can take on their health. Most people hide from depression or deny it. Worse yet, some even romanticize depression as the creative juice of great artists, or a cross to bear.[1] We can't afford to do this anymore because IT'S NOT HARMLESS TO BE DEPRESSED!

As you continue through the remainder of this book, you may feel upset and overwhelmed by all the possible harmful effects of depression. Don't despair. Depression is treatable. You can do something about it. Please keep this in mind.

We tend to think about depression as a purely emotional or psychological condition, divorced from the body or health in general. Actually, depression is a medical problem that is a risk factor for multiple health problems and premature death. Here are just some of the facts about depression you ought to know:

- Depression increases the chance of having a stroke.
- Depression increases the risk of having a heart attack and dying after one.
- Depression worsens chronic lung disease and diabetes.
- Depression makes chronic pain worse and harder to treat.
- Depression increases the risk of becoming obese. [2]
- Depression makes congestive heart failure and arthritis more disabling.
- Depression increases the likelihood that patients with chronic kidney disease will need dialysis.
- Depression nearly doubles the chance of getting Alzheimer's or Parkinson's disease.
- Depression weakens the immune system, making it harder to fight infection and increasing vulnerability to cancer.
- Depression increases the likelihood of needing long-term care. [3]
- Depression steepens the physical decline of aging, speeding loss of muscle strength and weakening balance and mobility. [4]
- Older persons with depression die sooner, from all causes, than those who are not depressed. Depression doubles the chance of dying over a two-year period.

To get a better feel for the connection of depression to these serious health problems, let's compare it to another disease that causes severe complications: diabetes. Without vigorous treatment, diabetes causes bodily damage that can result in blindness, heart and kidney disease, stroke, and amputations of the toes, feet, or legs. Depression has harmful effects on the body as well. While not everyone with diabetes takes care of it as carefully as they should, nearly all accept the need to do something about it, because they fear the complications. If you have depression, you need to take this disease just as seriously.

In earlier chapters we saw that depression is a serious brain disease. Beginning with this chapter and throughout part 2, we will look beyond depression as a disease of mental, emotional, and behavioral symptoms. We will see the scientific evidence of the wide-ranging impact depression has on physical health. I think you will conclude that the connection between depression and health is too strong to ignore, especially because the stakes are so high—your life. So, how does depression do it? There are two ways: behavior and physiology.

DEPRESSION, LIFESTYLE, BEHAVIOR, AND HEALTH

It's common sense that depressed individuals find it harder to take proper care of themselves. Let's consider the case of Jack in order to see how different symptom patterns of depression account for this.

Jack was a widowed, seventy-two-year-old retired bank manager. Jack had been on his own since his wife died five years earlier. His three children all lived out of state. Jack was fairly healthy, but he had type 2 diabetes. He also smoked three to four cigarettes per day.

Having been an excellent bank manager, managing his diabetes was right up Jack's alley. He had learned to cook meals using recipes in a diabetic cookbook. He exercised, watched his weight, limited alcohol consumption, took his diabetes pill faithfully, and checked his blood sugars daily. Then Jack developed depression, and things fell apart.

To this point, Jack's tale has been a true story. To give you an idea about how depression can pull the rug out from under someone like Jack, I've created three alternative scenarios, all borrowed from my experience with other patients.

Scenario 1

Jack's depression made him sad, hopeless, and pessimistic, and filled him with gloom-and-doom worries. He started drinking more in the evenings and, before long, started in the afternoon. Smoking more went along with the drinking, and soon Jack was up to a pack a day. He stopped exercising, began eating poorly, and took his medication erratically. Jack's blood sugars quickly crept up, and he felt so negative and depressed about this that he stopped checking them at all.

Scenario 2

Jack had depression-executive dysfunction syndrome, a pattern of late-life depression we reviewed in chapter 4. Depression left Jack feeling "blah," sluggish, down, and discouraged, and he was unmotivated and apathetic. As his depression worsened, Jack stopped exercising and started sleeping irregular hours. He rarely got up before midmorning. Jack decided it was too much trouble to check his blood sugar and ate either sugary children's cereal or leftover cold pizza for breakfast. He stopped using his cookbook to plan meals, did little grocery shopping, and mostly ate fast food, pizza, and doughnuts, when he ate at all. He no longer felt concerned about his diabetes and took his medication only when he remembered.

Scenario 3

Jack developed psychotic depression, which you may recall is a severe form of depression with irrational thoughts. As his depression got worse and worse, he began to have guilty thoughts that he was responsible for his wife's death. He became fixated on the idea that had he not been paying so much attention to taking care of his diabetes, he somehow would have known that his wife was about to have a fatal brain aneurysm and could have prevented it. He was terrified that his children would discover this and they would detest and disown him. He thought he was despicable and concluded that other patients with diabetes were more deserving of medication, so he stopped taking his pills.

Living a healthy lifestyle and managing an illness well, be it diabetes, chronic kidney disease, or high blood pressure, requires good executive skills. We reviewed the executive mental abilities in chapter 4. You may recall that these faculties are needed for planning and carrying out organized, goal-oriented behavior. It's no coincidence that high-level business managers are called executives, and you can appreciate how good Jack's executive abilities must have been before depression undid them in the second scenario.

To stay healthy you must also care about your well-being and have the energy and desire to care for yourself. Depressed persons who feel hopeless, negative, pessimistic, and down on themselves often do not. Some may not have the energy to manage their own care, or they may see their treatment as a futile rigmarole. Those who no longer care what happens to them, or even wish they were dead, lose all concern about the consequences of ignoring their treatment. If you think you would be better off dead, you probably do not care whether your blood pressure, blood sugar, or cholesterol is too high.

Depression turns conscientious, responsible individuals into lousy patients who take poor care of themselves. Depressed persons smoke and drink too much, eat poorly, fail to exercise, ignore their weight, take medication unreliably, and miss doctor appointments. And sometimes they outright refuse medical treatment that they would readily accept were they not depressed. When delusional depression causes irrational thinking, this is particularly apt to occur.

It is easy to see how such unhealthy behavior and lifestyle choices can cause patients with depression to get sicker and sicker and even die. Remarkably, though, these behavioral factors are only part of the picture. They do not fully explain the impact depression has on health. There is more to it.[5]

PHYSIOLOGY: DEPRESSION, STRESS, AND WEAR AND TEAR

I've referred to "physiology" a few times without defining it. So what is it? Physiology is a medical science dealing with how the body works. You have to understand how the body works in order to understand what has gone wrong in disease and how to treat it. To summarize chapters 2 and 3, you can think of depression as a disorder affecting the brain's physiology for emotions, thinking, and behavior. Now we'll look at depression's harmful affects on the body's physiology.

What does the tale of "Goldilocks and the Three Bears" have in common with physiology? The answer is that in both the importance of things being just right is the key. To remain healthy, our physiology must stay just right. Hearts, lungs, kidneys, and other organs require tightly controlled conditions to function normally. The brain is especially fussy. Examples of bodily functions that must stay just right include heart rate, core body temperature, blood pressure, blood sugar, and electrolyte levels. This narrow physiologic range is a kind of tightrope we all balance on.

Excess heat or cold; injury; starvation; dehydration; alcohol; sugary, fatty, and salty foods; pollution (including cigarette smoke); radiation; and infection are examples of physiologic stressors that buffet our bodies. Our physiology is designed to keep our core body temperature, blood pressure, blood sugar, electrolytes, and heart rate just right, but it can hold the line only so far. Any deviation of these parameters too far outside of the normal range can make us sick—we fall off the tightrope. How hard we get knocked off determines whether we fall into the safety net (doctor's office, hospital, or emergency room) or miss the net completely, and you can imagine what that means.

The stress response is the body's system for withstanding the many types of disturbances that can topple us from the tightrope. It is designed for immediate crises and challenges such as threats, disasters, injuries, illness, harsh environmental conditions, and emotional trauma and personal catastrophe. The nervous system, immune system, and hormonal systems do most of the heavy lifting in reacting to such stressors, including emotional stress. The brain is constantly on guard "watching" for internal and external stressors. When it senses a threat, it releases stress hormones, which, in turn, trigger various physiologic reactions, including a heightened state of inflammation throughout the body.

The stress response is designed to compensate for stressors that come and go. It works great in the short run, propping us up on the tightrope until things settle down, as long as they do so fairly soon. When stress is prolonged, its effects become destructive. Our bodies are not made for this.

An enormous amount of scientific research shows that depression produces a similar response to stress.[6] In chapter 2 we talked about the brain's emotional thermostat being turned up too high in depression. This state of overdrive in the brain triggers the stress response, which readies the heart, lungs, gastrointestinal system, immune system, and blood clotting systems for action. At the same time, the body's maintenance functions are shut down until the crisis passes. In effect, the brain runs the body ragged. The longer depression goes on, and the more often it occurs, the greater will be the accumulated wear and tear on the body.

Stress Hormones

Have you ever felt an adrenaline rush at a time of stress? Maybe you have experienced the adrenaline crash that occurs when prolonged stress at last comes to an end. In both stress and depression, the brain triggers a release of adrenaline and noradrenaline, two closely related stress hormones. These are also known as epinephrine and norepinephrine.

Adrenaline and noradrenaline get the body revved up to react to crises. Blood pressure and heart rate go up, and the lungs get ready to breathe harder. These hormones also set in motion a body-wide inflammatory reaction. Adrenaline and noradrenaline also destabilize the heart, electrically. This effect may explain how severe fright can trigger cardiac arrest.[7] Nothing so dramatic happens in depression, but the heart is left more vulnerable to irregular rhythms. The arteries in the heart become more prone to spasm, and the blood clots easier, a protective benefit during brief emergencies, but a harmful one if prolonged, as in depression. Enhanced blood clotting and heightened arterial spasm increase the chance of heart attacks.

The brain also triggers the release of cortisol, the other type of stress hormone, and a steroid. In response to stress, cortisol levels ordinarily rapidly increase and then quickly return to normal, once the stress subsides. But in depression, the normal shutoff doesn't work, and cortisol levels stay high. This effect is amplified with aging.

Cortisol helps when it goes up briefly, but when it remains high for longer periods it has harmful effects. These include weakened immunity to infection, high blood pressure, weight gain and obesity, osteoporosis, elevated blood sugar and resistance to insulin, poor wound healing, and damage to the brain.

Inflammation

Stress hormones set off a chain reaction releasing inflammatory agents known as cytokines. The cytokines cruise around the body inciting a widespread inflammatory state, including in the brain. This inflammatory state is an important first line of defense against infection, injury, and irritants. The inflammatory response attacks the problem but may cause local collateral damage to healthy tissue. In depression, these cytokines remain high, and the chronic inflammation causes widespread damage to the brain, blood vessels, intestines, heart, lungs, muscles, and bones.

Oxidative Damage

When the brain is in overdrive, during either stress or depression, energy for routine housekeeping activities is reduced. If this goes on very long, free radicals accumulate and cause oxidative damage. "Free radicals" and "oxidative damage" are terms you may have heard in relation to the aging process. But what do these terms, which sound as if they belong more in a chemistry book, actually mean?

Free radicals are chemical substances that cause oxidation, a chemical reaction. Rust is a familiar example of oxidation. You have certainly seen how rust can destroy iron-containing metals. Now, unless you are the tin man from the *Wizard of Oz*, you probably do not need to worry about rusting. But if oxidation can turn steel into rust, imagine how it can damage your proteins, chromosomes, DNA, muscles, joints, heart, lungs, and other organs, including, and especially, your brain, causing malfunction. So depression weakens the body's ability to neutralize free radicals and protect against the oxidative damage they cause.

BDNF Goes AWOL

BDNF stands for brain-derived neurotrophic factor. Now, there's a mouthful. BDNF is a protein that performs restorative, maintenance, and reparative actions in the brain. Normal levels of BDNF are essential for brain health and emotional well-being. The benefits of BDNF are not exclusive to the brain. BDNF also supports cardiovascular health and prevents obesity and diabetes. In depression, levels of BDNF are abnormally low. Ordinarily, BDNF might check the damaging effects of stress hormones, inflammation, and oxidative damage. During states of depression, BDNF is not up to the task.

DEPRESSION CAN MAKE YOU OLD BEFORE YOUR TIME

Let's consider the repeated head injuries that professional boxers and football players sustain as a model for the damage depression can do to the body. Repeated blows to the head, over many bouts, can give prizefighters a form of dementia called chronic traumatic encephalopathy. It's beginning to look as though the same thing happens to professional football players who have their bells rung (hits to the head) too many times. The repeated blows to these athletes' heads stresses their brains, giving some of them dementia in middle age. Their brains share more in common with those of eighty-year-old Alzheimer's patients than healthy middle-aged adults. In this sense, these athletes' brains have become old before their time.

Depression has much the same effect. Head trauma stresses the brain mechanically, and depression stresses the brain physiologically. Each episode of depression in life is akin to another "hit." The physiologic wear and tear from each salvo of stress hormones, inflammation, and oxidation adds up. A single prolonged or very severe episode of depression is probably just as bad. When enough is enough, organs may start to break down, age-related diseases become more common, and health declines. Depressed persons effectively become old before their time.

Have you ever torn your rotator cuff? It is a common injury, and I have many patients that have done this from falling. Suppose you did it from a nasty fall skiing when you were younger. With time and proper care, it may have healed well. It would have healed much faster and more completely when you were younger because aging weakens the reparative and restorative capacity of the body. But now consider this. Now that you are older, to the eyes of a trained orthopedic surgeon, your previously injured shoulder might look older than your other shoulder. The wear and tear from the prior injury effectively aged your shoulder faster than the uninjured one. Depression increases the wear and tear on your brain and body.

WHEN YOUR TELOMERES' NUMBERS ARE UP, SO IS YOURS

If you think about all the health problems associated with depression that I listed at the beginning of this chapter, you'll notice they are all conditions associated with aging. Older people are much more likely to have these conditions than are younger people. Because depression seems to bring these conditions on sooner, researchers have suggested that depression causes a state of accelerated aging.[8]

How do we really know that depression causes accelerated aging? The answer is that telomeres don't lie. Aging research has zeroed in more and more on telomeres.

Telomeres are molecular caps on the DNA, the substance in cells that contains all a person's genes. They are like aglets, the caps on the ends of shoelaces that prevent unraveling. Telomeres protect DNA from damage during cell division. Scientists can measure the length of telomeres. Each time a cell divides, its telomeres shorten. The shortening of telomeres is a measure of an organism's age, because cells divide only so many times in their lifespan. When a cell's telomeres shorten below a critical length, the cell becomes susceptible to breakdown, illness, and death. As more cells succumb to this fate, organs begin to show signs of aging and become prone to disease.

Our bodies have physiologic tools to keep our telomeres from shortening too fast. Exercise makes telomeres longer. That is the good news. The bad news is that chronic stress and depression speeds the shortening of telomeres. The more cumulative depression a person has throughout life, the shorter their telomeres.[9] The degree of shortening of telomeres seen in persons with depression suggests that depression has aged them five years or more, literally making them old before their time. Telomere length may represent the smoking gun that implicates depression in declining health and premature death.

DON'T SHOOT CRAPS WITH YOUR HEALTH

We all like certainty and seek predictability in our lives. We all want to know what things will or won't make us sick. Unfortunately, in medicine, there are few certainties, just probabilities. Healthcare professionals deal with risk factors, and you need to as well.

Risk factors are things that increase the chance of getting ill or dying. Smoking, high blood pressure, and elevated cholesterol are risk factors for stroke and heart disease, and so is depression. There are two types of risk factors: those you can't do anything about and those you can. Genes are an example of the first type of risk factors. If you have the genes for a disease, there is nothing you can do to change that. Other risk factors are modifiable, meaning you can do something about them.

You can quit smoking, lose weight, lower your cholesterol, and take medications for your blood pressure.

Depression is a modifiable risk factor for disease and premature death. If you have depression, your chances of a range of diseases and dying younger are greater. You can lower your risk by having treatment for depression. If you have depression and don't get help for it, you are gambling your health away with dice loaded against you. You may not roll craps every time, but you will more often than you should, and you'll eventually go bust. Treatment for depression swaps the loaded dice for a fair set, which greatly improves your odds of staying healthy and living longer.

CONCLUSION

Depression is a brain disease that runs the body ragged, causing heightened wear and tear, increased illness, and premature death. The shortening of telomeres seen in depression leads to the frightening conclusion that depression accelerates aging. The good news is that you can do something about depression. Treatment works. In the coming chapters of part 2, we will look more closely at depression's impact on individual health problems. In each chapter we will see that treatment of depression can restore mental and emotional wellness and also improve health, independence, and life expectancy. You can take action to improve your health and live longer.

6

WHEN HEARTACHE CAUSES HEART "ACHE"

Depression and Heart Disease

Sometime during the next year, your doctor may test your cholesterol, blood sugar, and vitamin D levels to make sure they are normal. If you are a woman, you may have a Pap smear to look for signs of cervical cancer, or a mammogram to check for breast cancer. And if you see an ophthalmologist, he or she will check the pressure in your eyes to make sure you do not have glaucoma. These are examples of screening tests healthcare professionals routinely order for their patients. The goal of screening is to catch disease early, before it has a chance to cause serious health problems.

Questions about exercise, diet, smoking, and alcohol consumption; measurements of blood pressure and weight; and tests for diabetes and high cholesterol are widely used screens for cardiovascular disease— with good reason. According to the Centers for Disease Control and Prevention (CDC), heart disease is the leading cause of death and disability in the United States. Coronary artery disease is the most common cause of death from heart disease. There are over seven hundred thousand heart attacks per year.[1] Doctors use the information from screening tests to help their patients prevent illness and stay healthy. Depending on which screens are positive, they might recommend diet, exercise, quitting smoking, or cutting down on drinking; they might also prescribe medications for high blood pressure, elevated cholesterol, or diabetes.

Depression is very common among those with heart disease. That may not surprise you, but you probably didn't know that depression is a risk factor for serious heart disease. In fact, depression was recently added to the list of risk factors for heart disease, on par with smoking and high blood pressure.

THE CASE OF THOMAS

Thomas was a sixty-seven-year-old former bus driver. A smoker since the age of seventeen, Thomas had tried to quit five or six times. At sixty-two, Thomas developed coronary artery disease and had two stents put in. Stents are mesh tubes placed inside blocked sections of coronary arteries to keep them open. This scared Thomas into cutting down his smoking to a pack a week.

Two years later, though, Thomas developed depression. Smoking helped him feel a little better, at least briefly, and he gradually increased to a pack per day. Abusing a substance, be it cigarettes, marijuana, or alcohol, is never a good way to deal with depression, or any other problem.

Because of his health problems, Thomas decided to retire. He had a decent pension and few worries, but being retired made Thomas more depressed. He felt lost, without purpose. His cardiologist advised Thomas to get some exercise, but he became even more sedentary. Then he had a heart attack.

Fortunately, Thomas's heart attack was not a very big one. But days later, in the coronary care unit (CCU), he had periods of dangerously abnormal heart rhythms. He was also extremely depressed and felt hopeless. Thomas's cardiologist was worried and wanted Thomas to see a psychiatrist about taking an antidepressant medication, but Thomas declined. Talking to a "shrink" was not his "bag." And his wife discouraged it. She had read, on the Internet, that antidepressants are not safe for cardiac patients.

On the fifth day Thomas's heart went into a life-threatening rhythm called ventricular fibrillation, and he suffered a cardiac arrest. The team did everything they could to bring him back, but after an hour, Thomas was gone. The cause of death was cardiac arrest, but on that day depression killed Thomas as much as heart disease did. Let's see how.

DEPRESSION IS A CARDIAC RISK FACTOR

Depression is a risk factor for developing heart disease no different from high cholesterol, smoking, high blood pressure, diabetes, and inactivity. Here are some important factors to be aware of:

- Depression doubles the rate of coronary artery disease among the elderly.[2]
- Depression is a slightly greater risk for heart disease than is smoking or high blood pressure. Only diabetes is a greater risk.[3]
- If you already have coronary artery disease, and you undergo coronary artery bypass surgery, depression doubles or triples your chance of dying.
- Depression affects 45 percent of patients after a heart attack.[4]
- After a heart attack, depression increases the chance of cardiac complications. It quadruples the chance of dying within four months and doubles the chance of dying of heart disease within five years.[5]
- One in three patients with congestive heart failure have depression. Depression makes congestive heart failure worse and increases the chance of dying from congestive heart failure.[6]

The evidence for the role of depression in heart disease is so strong that the American Heart Association did a remarkable thing in 2014. It added depression to the list of risk factors for which cardiologists and other doctors should screen their patients. They put depression on the list of things that are bad for the heart, smack at the top of the list with smoking.

CORONARY ARTERY DISEASE 101

Let's look at what the heart does and how heart disease affects it, so we can appreciate the impact of depression. The heart pumps blood throughout the body, supplying all the organs, including the brain, with oxygen and nutrients. Four heart chambers, made of specialized cardiac muscle, do the pumping. The chambers fill with blood and then squeeze it out, creating the pumping action. Think of an uncapped tube of toothpaste. Imagine how the toothpaste would squirt out if you grabbed it with both hands and quickly squeezed as tightly as you could.

The heart works hard and must pump blood into itself as well to meet its own demands for oxygen and nutrients. The coronary arteries route some of the blood exiting the heart right back into the heart muscle. In coronary artery disease, the coronary arteries become clogged by plaque, a process called atherosclerosis. Depression increases the chance of this happening.

If the coronary arteries are partially blocked, blood still gets through but not enough. When greater demands are put on the heart, by walking up stairs, for example, chest pain, known as angina, may occur. Angina is a sign that the heart is not getting enough oxygen to do the work required of it.

If the plaque in a coronary artery cracks, frays, or gets roughed up, then, as the blood flows past it, a clot may form. Such a clot can completely block off the coronary artery. A spasm of the coronary arteries also reduces blood flow through them. Stress and depression can increase spasms. When blood flow to part of the heart is too severely interrupted, a heart attack occurs.

To visualize this, imagine the rain gutters on a house. If you live in a northern climate, you may see where I am going. In autumn, when the leaves fall off the trees, some of them get caught in the gutters, where they accumulate, something like plaque. When it rains, the water will wash the leaves right into the downspout, and they will flow out onto the ground. No problem. But all it takes is for a small twig to get caught in the downspout opening to catch the leaves as they flow past, starting a "clot." The wet leaves build up, eventually blocking the downspout completely, and water comes to a standstill in the gutters, until it spills over onto the side of your house. What a mess! Climbing up a ladder on a cold autumn day to clear a blockage of wet leaves is no fun.

During a heart attack, the section of the heart supplied by the blocked artery gets no blood. Without emergency medical treatment to open the blood flow in the blocked coronary artery, the affected piece of the heart muscle will die. If enough of the heart is damaged, its pumping action will be weakened. Depression also increases the chance of this happening.

The heart's four chambers must pump in sequence for the heart to circulate the blood properly. The rhythmic pumping of the heart is coordinated, electrically, by circuits in the heart. Picture an ancient Roman galley. I'm sure you have an idea about these from movies you've seen. Usually they are depicted with slaves chained to their oars rowing to the beat of a drummer. The heart's electrical circuits bang its "drum" so that all the heart muscle cells contract at the right time making the chambers pump. The heart's electrical circuits are under the control of the nervous system. Just as the galley's captain tells the drummer how fast to beat it, signals from the brain affect the heart's circuits.

Damage to the heart can directly disrupt these electrical circuits, affecting the heart's rhythm. Injury to the heart muscle itself can leave it electrically unstable, vulnerable to irregular rhythms and even cardiac arrest. The high levels of stress hormones present during depression also destabilize the heart electrically, producing the same effects. Without a drumbeat in our imaginary galley, the slaves will row willy-nilly, if they row at all, and the boat will become dead in the water. When the equivalent of this happens in the heart, it is called ventricular fibrillation. When "V-fib" occurs, the heart must immediately be defibrillated—jump-started back into action—or death occurs. Depression also increases the chance of these things happening. This is what happened to Thomas, and he died.

Congestive heart failure (CHF) is a more gradual, less dramatic result of coronary artery disease. The poor circulation of blood through the coronary arteries over a long time eventually weakens the heart muscle, and the pumping action of the heart fails. When this occurs, blood is circulated around the body too slowly. Patients with CHF begin to feel tired, sluggish, or lethargic. Fluid backs up throughout the body. The telltale signs are swelling in the feet and ankles, and shortness of breath due to fluid in the lungs.

I like to explain to my patients that congestive heart failure is akin to living in a house with a very wet basement and a worn-out sump pump that doesn't do the job. There are a lot of damp basements in my area. Heavy rains flood the basement until the homeowners spring for a new sump pump. Many of my patients are fixed-income retirees living on

Social Security, so food and medicine usually are higher priorities in their budgets. If you live in a region plagued by historic droughts, I apologize for all the analogies to problems of excessive water. Similar to the worn-out sump pump, the heart in congestive heart failure also doesn't do a good enough job, which means the body, including the brain and the heart, does not get the circulation it needs. And depression makes this condition worse, too. Now let's see how depression does these things to the heart.

BEHAVIOR AND PHYSIOLOGY

As I described in chapter 5, behavior and physiology are the primary ways depression harms the body, including the heart.

Let's start with behavior. Preventing heart disease and its complications involves adopting a heart-healthy lifestyle. It's not easy to do this when you are depressed. Actually, it's tough enough for many who are not depressed. If you have ever tried to lose weight, exercise more, or quit smoking, then you can imagine how insurmountable depression can make such tasks seem. Thomas illustrates the difficulty and what often happens instead. He failed to exercise and quit smoking and instead became less active and smoked more. Depressed patients also have a tougher time sticking to low-salt, low-fat diets. Those with diabetes may ignore their diabetic diets. And it is harder to be faithful about taking blood pressure and cholesterol medications when you have depression. Finally, heart attack survivors with depression make a poor effort in cardiac rehab. Studies bear out that depression's biggest impact on heart disease is through behavioral effects.[7] But behavioral effects are not the whole story.

Physiology takes a backseat to behavior in heart disease, but it nonetheless plays an important role, and a far more complicated one. You may recall from the previous chapter that stress hormones, inflammation, and oxidative damage are depression's henchmen. The heart is a sitting-duck target for these toxic effects. Elevated levels of adrenaline and noradrenaline make the heart beat faster, and elevated cortisol raises blood pressure. This double whammy piles extra work on the heart that it can't afford to do. Inflammation and oxidative damage irritate the inner lining of the coronary arteries making heart attack–causing clots more likely. At the same time, depression makes the platelets, the elements in blood that form clots, more prone to stick together, and it increases the levels of clotting factors in the blood. This is a recipe for disaster.

The greater clotting tendency in depression heightens the risk of not only a heart attack but also a stroke. We'll get to strokes, the other scourge of cardiovascular disease, in the next chapter. Remarkably, successful treatment of depression returns blood clotting to normal.

And finally, as I described earlier, depression makes the heart electrically unstable. Adrenaline and noradrenaline are once again to blame. As I described in the previous chapter, depression causes heightened levels of these stress hormones to circulate throughout the entire body. The increased action of these stress hormones makes the heart electrically unstable and prone to cardiac arrest. But their effects in heart disease may have less to do with the higher circulating levels of these hormones and more to do with direct effects through the brain-heart connection.[8]

The heart is directly "wired" to the brain via the nervous system, a connection called the brain-heart connection. In emergencies, this helps the heart respond immediately to demands put on it by the brain. For example, if you sense danger and start to run, your heart must start beating faster right away. Your heart can't afford to wait for the "snail mail" of the circulation for delivery of the needed stress hormones. It needs a cell-phone instant message. The brain-heart connection does this through direct connections between the brain and the heart. No doubt this allows us to escape any number of life-threatening jams. It also makes athletic activity possible. But it also leaves the heart more sensitive to unhealthy emotional states and opens us up to the possibility of literally being scared to death.[9] In depression, a brain on overdrive runs the heart ragged.

TREATMENT OF DEPRESSION AND HEART HEALTH

If you smoke and want to save your heart, you need to quit. Everybody gets this. If you have depression, it is just as important to have treatment for it. Few people realize this, but the American Heart Association has done a good job getting the word out, at least to cardiologists.

Treatment of depressed cardiac patients with antidepressant medications reduces further cardiac problems and saves lives.[10] I firmly believe this, having seen it time and again in my thirty years of practicing geriatric psychiatry. But simply being on an antidepressant medication or having psychotherapy does little good. In one study, patients who received treatment for depression that didn't work had more than double the risk of further cardiac events (dying or having to be rehospitalized for heart problems) than patients whose depression got better. To help reduce heart disease, treatment of depression must be effective.[11]

ARE ANTIDEPRESSANT MEDICATIONS SAFE FOR PATIENTS WITH HEART DISEASE?

When I began my medical career in the 1980s, doctors believed it was safe to give cardiac patients antidepressants. They were not as risky as was widely thought and could be used to treat many cardiac patients, as long as extra precautions were taken. Tofranil, Pamelor, Elavil, and Sinequan are examples of tricyclic antidepressants with which older readers may be familiar.

There is even less cause for concern with the new antidepressant medications available today. The selective serotonin reuptake inhibitors (or SSRIs, such as Prozac, Paxil, Celexa, and Zoloft), venlafaxine (Effexor), bupropion (Wellbutrin), and mirtazapine (Remeron) are all safe for the heart. Unfortunately, word gets out slowly. I still encounter cardiologists and other specialists who continue to believe that antidepressant medications are unsafe for patients with heart disease.

Unfortunately, fear about the safety of antidepressants for the heart was stoked in 2011 when the Food and Drug Administration (FDA) issued a warning about the use of the antidepressant citalopram (Celexa) in certain vulnerable patients. This medication, an SSRI, is almost always safe and is often a good medication for older adults with anxiety or depression. But citalopram can very rarely cause a fatal heart rhythm abnormality in persons with a condition called QT prolongation, or those vulnerable to get it. QT prolongation is easy to spot on an electrocardiogram, making it possible to take precautions and prevent serious problems. The FDA dealt with this risk by lowering the maximum approved dose for citalopram. The warning reinforced fear of cardiac side effects of antidepressant medications and once again made some doctors and patients—Thomas's wife had heard about this—skittish about all antidepressants.

I understand their concerns. Doctors should be cautious. And patients with heart disease should be careful. But here's the thing. If you have heart disease and depression, you should be much, much more concerned about depression. Depression is a far greater risk than are antidepressant medications, which actually may be your ticket to a healthier life, as long as they are prescribed and monitored carefully, by a doctor with the necessary expertise.

DO YOU NEED TO SEE A PSYCHIATRIST?

Many patients with heart disease have a cardiologist, but few have a psychiatrist, and some may not have access to one. What if your cardiologist wants to prescribe antidepressant medications for you? Should you let him or her do so? In general this is a good thing, so the answer is yes. Cardiologists have all the tools at their disposal to monitor the safety of antidepressants for your heart. Most of them will do a good job, as long as they make a correct diagnosis of depression and use antidepressant medications effectively. Here are a few tips to help you make sure this happens.

First, remember the importance of correct diagnosis. One way to screen for depression is with depression symptom questionnaires that healthcare professionals sometimes have patients fill out. Based on the American Heart Association recommendations I mentioned earlier, cardiologists will hopefully be doing more and more of this. These questionnaires are a good start. I even use them in my practice. But answers on a questionnaire alone are not enough to diagnose depression, whether the questionnaire is two questions long or thirty. As we saw in chapter 4, much more is involved in diagnosing depression correctly. So don't accept treatment for depression based only on your answers to a questionnaire.

If you have depression and are already receiving treatment, the second thing you can do is make sure the treatment works. Many patients with depression are correctly diagnosed and given the right treatment, but they do not get better. The problem is that a low starting dose is begun, which is a good thing, but then the antidepressant is not increased to the point at which the depression improves. Patients being treated for depression must be watched closely to make sure they are improving, and the treatment must be adjusted if they are not. IF YOU ARE NOT GETTING BETTER, IT'S UP TO YOU TO LET YOUR DOCTOR KNOW THIS AND MAKE IT CLEAR THAT YOU EXPECT SOMETHING MORE TO BE DONE.

And third, if you are getting nowhere, consider having a consultation with a psychiatrist. Try to find one who is knowledgeable about treating patients with heart disease. If you are an older adult, geriatric psychiatrists have the expertise you need.

CONCLUSION: THE HEART OF THE MATTER

Living with depression instead of getting treatment for it increases your risk of heart disease. Don't do it. If you already have heart disease and you get depression as well, which happens a lot, things can become even worse. Heart disease can spoil a happy retirement with pain, functional limitations, and worse. Treating depression improves your odds substantially. No one should let himself or herself live with untreated depression. This treatment may be as critical as any of the other steps your cardiologist takes to keep you healthy. Your heart depends on it.

7

TREATMENT OF DEPRESSION MAY BE A STROKE OF LUCK

Depression and Stroke

If you read chapter 6, you not only learned about coronary artery disease but also know something about stroke. The reason I can say this is that heart attack and stroke share something in common: they are the evil twins of cardiovascular disease.

Much of what we know about depression as a risk for coronary artery disease and cardiac complications after a heart attack applies to stroke. If you skipped the last chapter because you were eager to delve into stroke, don't worry. You'll catch up quickly. To boil it down, if you have heart disease due to poor circulation, chances are you also have brain disease due to poor circulation. They go hand in hand. And depression plays a similar role in both.

Remember Sydney A and Sydney B from the "Tale of Two Sydneys" in the introduction to this book? Each man was waylaid by a stroke that neither saw coming. In both cases, stroke triggered post-stroke depression. In chapter 3, we learned that stroke does this by damaging mood circuits in the brain. In Sydney B's case we also saw how post-stroke depression, left untreated, triggered a downward spiral of declining health, nursing home care, and premature death. In this chapter we will look at the flip side of depression and stroke: how depression can cause stroke.

UNHAPPY JULIETTE: A TICKING TIME BOMB

Juliette was sixty-two years old when she sought my help. She was fairly young for my practice. The overwhelming majority of patients who see geriatric specialists, me included, are older, usually seventy-five and over. I saw Juliette because she had problems that had made her old before her time. She needed my help and had nowhere else to turn.

Tragic, and so unnecessary, are the bylines to Juliette's story. Juliette came from a good family and had a happy childhood. She went to college; became a journalist; married a kind, earnest fellow, named Ron; and raised two well-adjusted children, who were themselves thriving. It sounds like a charmed life.

The black clouds drifted in even before Juliette graduated from college. Unlike her friends, who were eager and idealistic, Juliette couldn't see the point to anything—education, career, or family life. A chronic pessimism set in. She became a gloomy, negative, and dour person. Others found her to be a wet blanket who always saw the glass as half empty. Juliette's husband was an eternally enthusiastic, cheerful optimist, and the marriage worked somehow. Marriage, children, home life, and work were okay, but nothing was good. Life was drab and gray, devoid of bright colors, joy, or pleasure. She was "just going through the motions," and the future seemed full of nothing but drudgery capped off by sickness and death. Juliette had dysthymia.

You may recall that dysthymia, also called persistent depressive disorder, is a form of low-grade, chronic depression. Because dysthymia is not usually as severely disabling as major depressive disorder, persons with dysthymia often just live with it, suffering year after year, without seeking treatment. This aspect makes dysthymia even more harmful to health than more serious forms of depression, for which people are more likely to get help.

Live with it is exactly what Juliette did. She didn't smoke or drink, and somehow managed to keep her weight down, but she didn't eat a well-balanced diet and never exercised. Everyone she knew got used to her negative, grim attitude. They dismissed it as "Juliette being Juliette." Not a single person suggested she get professional help. All who were close to her thought "that's just how she is."

Juliette developed type 2 diabetes in her late fifties. In the next chapter we will see that depression might have brought this on. Diabetes was not too much of an emotional setback for Juliette. A once-a-day pill was all that she needed to keep her blood sugar under control. And being the pessimistic person that she was, she had been expecting her health to give way. Turning sixty years old was more unsettling to Juliette, and to family members it seemed like a turning point: she became more and more depressed thereafter.

At a time in her life when Juliette might have been able to enjoy the fruits of marriage, parenthood, and career, she saw nothing good ahead. Her depression deepened further, and she decided to retire early. Juliette sat home with nothing to do. Many days she didn't get dressed. Most mornings she awoke by three o'clock and lay awake in bed consumed by the thought that life was over and it had been pointless. Facing each day filled her with dread. Juliette now had major depression.

Ron and the children thought Juliette ought to get professional help, but they didn't know what kind was best. It didn't matter, though, because Juliette refused to consider it. She didn't see the point. She'd always felt this way about life and now was getting old. How was that supposed to make her happier? She procrastinated.

Then disaster struck. One morning Juliette woke up feeling strange. She struggled to get out of bed and promptly fell. The right side of her body didn't seem to work properly. She decided to call one of her children but could not remember either of their names. She knew how to dial 9-1-1, but when the operator came on Juliette was unable to speak. Juliette had suffered a stroke.

Somehow an ambulance came and took Juliette to the hospital. A blood clot had formed in the carotid artery on the left side of her neck, broken off, and flowed into her head, where it blocked the circulation to the left side of her brain. All the doctors could do was start anticoagulant medications (often called blood thinners) to prevent further clots from forming.

Juliette spent five days in the hospital and then six weeks in a nursing home rehabilitation program. She improved slightly. She could express basic needs in short sentences, feed herself, and stand and walk with assistance.

You may recall that strokes in the left frontal lobe of the brain of right-handed people often cause depression. Juliette had already been depressed, and this stroke certainly didn't make her any better. The nurses and physical therapists noticed the depression right away, and the nursing home doctor prescribed 50 mg of the antidepressant medication sertraline (Zoloft). Ron was pleased that something was finally being done for Juliette's depression, and he asked Juliette's primary care doctor to continue the medication after she returned home.

Three months went by without any improvement. Juliette was anguished, cried all the time, and became totally helpless. Within days of returning home, she stopped doing her physical therapy. A physical therapist came to her home, but after the second visit she refused to answer the door. She stopped doing things the therapists told Ron she could easily do herself. Mostly she sat in a dark room with the shades drawn and appeared to have given up. That was when Juliette's primary care doctor referred her to me.

When I met Juliette she was profoundly sad, gloomy, and hopeless. It was painful to watch her struggle to get the words out, but she conveyed a feeling of uselessness and worthlessness. She thought her life was over, had no desire to go on living, and wished the stroke had finished her. I raised the dose of the sertraline to 75 mg, and three weeks later she started to improve. As we will see in chapter 21, it's not usually that easy, but in Juliette's case it was.

Three months later Juliette was much better. She stopped crying, smiled and laughed naturally at times, and tried to do more things for herself. She developed a desire to get better and became determined to help herself. One year later, she could walk with a cane, dress herself, and read children's books aloud to her grandchildren. Her speech was halting at times, and her grandchildren thought she sounded funny, but Juliette was able to make a reading game out of it, and they had fun. To everyone's surprise and joy, Juliette was enjoying family life and looking forward to things. Two years after her stroke, Juliette was able to speak well enough to carry on a fairly fluent conversation. She didn't need my help any longer, and I have not seen her since.

STROKE IS A GAME CHANGER

The scariest thing about strokes is that they strike suddenly, often without warning. Talk about having the rug pulled out from under you. Stroke is a true scourge of aging that can abruptly turn a happy retirement into an old age marred by physical and mental disability. In one fell swoop, a stroke can make a healthy, vigorous older adult old before his or her time.

Try to imagine what it might be like to find yourself helpless and completely dependent upon others. How about if you could not communicate with those around you? You know exactly what you want to say, but the words will not come out. Or maybe you can speak, but everything you say is gibberish, and others make no sense to you. What about not being able to feel or move one side of your body? How would you cope with not being able to walk, dress yourself, feed yourself, shower, or use the toilet on your own? This is some of the horror of a stroke.

According to the Centers for Disease Control and Prevention, nearly 800,000 people have a stroke every year in the United States, and 130,000 of them die. Two-thirds of strokes strike people over age sixty-five. Stroke is the fourth leading cause of death in the United States.[1]

The National Stroke Association lists high blood pressure, atrial fibrillation, diabetes, elevated cholesterol, carotid artery disease, diet, inactivity, and alcohol abuse as risk factors for stroke.[2] Have you noticed the overlap with risks for heart disease? This list makes up the common cardiovascular risk factors and illustrates the rule of thumb I alluded to in the beginning: "What's bad for the heart is bad for the brain," and vice versa. Did you also notice that depression is not included in the National Stroke Association's list of stroke risk factors? It ought to be.

WHAT IS A STROKE?

Before we go any farther, let's define stroke a little better. You may hear a stroke referred to as a cerebrovascular accident, CVA for short. We doctors love long, complicated names, especially if we can abbreviate them with initials. You will hear many types of doctors say "CVA" except neurologists. Neurologists, specialists in nervous system diseases, and the ones with the expertise to diagnose and treat stroke, tend to call it "stroke." I prefer the name stroke also and will use it in this book. Just keep in mind that when you hear people refer to a CVA they are talking about a stroke. They mean the same thing.

I have always thought it odd to call a stroke an accident. There's nothing accidental about it. It's not as if a bee flew into someone's car while they were driving and stung them on the nose causing them to run a red light and rear-end you. That's an accident. A stroke is not accidental—disastrous, yes, but accidental, no. And, more to the point, if you have smoked or ignored high blood pressure, diabetes, or depression, and have a stroke, "cerebrovascular negligence" seems more apt, because you might have prevented that stroke and spared yourself and your family a whole lot of misery.

Think of stroke as a heart attack in the brain, or a "brain attack." Sudden interruption of the circulation in one or more of the arteries in the brain causes stroke. Blood flow can be cut off by either a blockage, often caused by a clot, or bleeding. Strokes due to blockages make up the vast majority. Strokes also vary in severity from very mild to catastrophically severe, and many are fatal.

The areas of the brain that lose circulation immediately stop working. The symptoms of a stroke reflect the loss of the functions the affected brain area performs. If circulation is restored quickly, the symptoms pass. But if circulation does not resume quickly, the parts of the brain involved die. Some patients regain the lost functions fully, others not at all, and many somewhere in between. What improvement takes place may happen within days to weeks, but more often it requires months to years. Symptoms of strokes include weakness; paralysis or loss of feeling, usually affecting one side of the body; slurred speech; trouble swallowing; difficulty speaking; impaired comprehension; double vision; staggering; numbness or loss of feeling; and confusion—and, of course, depression.

DEPRESSION CAUSES STROKE

As we have already seen, stroke often causes depression. But the opposite also is true: depression causes stroke. And depression interferes with recovery from stroke. The link between depression and stroke has been the subject of many studies done in many countries involving a variety of patients with depression. The bottom line is that after the effects of other conditions that cause stroke, such as smoking, heart disease, diabetes, and high blood pressure, are factored out, the cumulative data indicate that depression on its own increases the chance of having a stroke by 30 to 50 percent. This makes depression as great a risk for stroke as is smoking![3] Depression and smoking are alike in another important way; both are preventable causes of stroke. You can quit smoking, and you can get treatment for depression.

A finding from one study is especially alarming. Researchers found that the risk from depression is higher the younger you are. Depression poses a greater risk for stroke for persons in their fifties and early sixties than those in their seventies and eighties.[4] So if you are younger than sixty-five years old and have depression, don't assume that stroke is something you do not have to worry about for many years. It may be lurking right outside your door, and you cannot afford to put off getting treatment for depression, as Juliette did.

HOW DOES DEPRESSION CAUSE STROKE?

Scientists do not know for sure how depression causes stroke. Behavior and physiology, now familiar suspects, are the likely culprits.

First, let's look at behavior. If you have read the previous two chapters, then you are familiar with the concept that people with depression do not take as good care of themselves as they would if they did not have depression. We will see this apply again and again throughout the rest of this book. Depression sufferers become lackadaisical about treatment for high blood pressure, elevated cholesterol, and diabetes. They lapse into unhealthy eating habits, smoke more, drink excessively, and give up exercising. These behavioral patterns increase the risks for both coronary artery disease and stroke. Let's face it, many people are not so good about these things at their best, and they neglect themselves even more when they have depression.

On top of these lifestyle and behavioral effects are the physiological effects. As I said before, stroke and coronary artery disease are both circulatory conditions. In each case, damage to an organ occurs when part of its circulation is blocked. Arteries become blocked when damage to their linings stimulates the formation of clots. In some cases of stroke, these clots block the artery where they form. In other cases, pieces of a clot break off and flow downstream in the artery, eventually blocking it off like a cork in the neck of a wine bottle.

As we have learned already, depression brings about heightened levels of stress hormones, inflammation, and oxidative damage, all of which damage the inner linings of arteries. Just as this happens in the heart, it can happen in the brain. Platelets, the clotting elements in blood that are the first line of defense against bleeding, are prone to stick to areas of irritation in arteries. Depression also makes the platelets more prone to clump together in clots. The medical term for such clots is thrombus. Depression thus creates "a perfect storm" for the type of thrombus formation that causes stroke.

DEPRESSION AFTER A STROKE

It's bad enough that depression can bring on a stroke. After a stroke, depression can make things worse. Depression worsens recovery from a stroke. And depression increases the chance of having another stroke.

In the minutes, hours, and days after a stroke, emergency medical care is most needed. Once the crisis passes, the emphasis shifts to rehabilitation. Each stroke victim's potential to recover is different. The recovery of lost functions can range from nearly complete to none at all. Some stroke patients recover quickly, but others take months or years, if they recover at all.

Patients with post-stroke depression do not recover as quickly or as much. Stroke patients who have depression become more disabled with the passage of time after their stroke. Their ability to care for themselves declines, and they become more cognitively impaired. Some become frankly demented.[5] How does depression do this? The answer, again, is behavior and physiology.

The brain damage caused by a stroke is permanent. There is no cure. But the brain does have a limited ability to repair itself. Dead brain cells are lost for good, but the surrounding cells can form new and more extensive connections, essentially rerouting functions around the damage. This ability is called neuroplasticity, a long and complicated word, but one that spells hope for stroke survivors. I think "neuroplasticity" is a word you will hear more about in the years to come in news media covering breakthroughs in the treatment of Alzheimer's disease, traumatic brain injury, stroke, and other disabling brain diseases.

Neuroplasticity isn't limited to existing brain cells forming new connections. It also includes the appearance of new brain cells in certain areas of the brain to replace older ones that have died. This constant turnover of brain cells and the formation of new connections are both essential for good mental health. Neuroplasticity allows the brain to change or remodel itself slightly and provides a means for the brain to compensate for damage.

Brain-derived neurotrophic factor, BDNF for short, is a protein with a key role in promoting neuroplasticity. Without BDNF, neuroplasticity doesn't work. You may recall from chapter 5 that depression shuts off BDNF. Stroke recovery depends greatly on BDNF. One likely possibility is that depression interferes with stroke recovery by shutting off BDNF.

Stroke rehab takes much more than sitting around watching television while you wait for BDNF to work its magic. Behavior matters as much. The stroke victim must make a significant personal investment in physical therapy. Progress occurs in small steps, which must be practiced and repeated over and over again. Motivation, effort, determination, discipline, grit, and hope are needed as much as BDNF, if not more. These traits tend to be in short supply among those with depression.

I often see the impact depression has on stroke rehab in my practice. Juliette, Sydney A, and Sydney B are just three examples. I have lost count of how many other patients I've treated for depression after a stroke. I've seen them bemoan their fate but make little effort in their therapy. It's especially hard on family members, who stand by helplessly, getting more and more frustrated, upset, and discouraged.

Fortunately, treatment of depression makes a difference. In fact, I can tell that my depressed stroke patients are starting to respond to their antidepressant medication when they begin to show interest in their physical therapy again.

IN MEDICINE, LIGHTNING CAN STRIKE TWICE IN THE SAME PLACE

The possibility of having a stroke is depressing. If you've already had one stroke, here's a terrifying thought: you could have another. One in four Americans who have a stroke will have another one during the rest of their life. For many this may not be that far off. Within five years of a stroke, 24 percent of women and 42 percent of men will experience a second stroke. One-fourth of the eight hundred thousand strokes that occur each year in the United States occur in someone who has already had a stroke.[6] By now you shouldn't be surprised that depression doesn't help this situation either. After a stroke, depression shortens the time until another stroke.[7] I share this information with patients who are reluctant to have psychiatric treatment. Sometimes they find it convincing and compelling, and it helps them feel less reluctant to be treated for depression. They still want to avoid psychiatry like the plague, but they want to avoid another stroke even more.

TREATMENT OF DEPRESSION IN STROKE VICTIMS

As it does in heart disease, treatment of depression addresses risk factors for stroke and reduces the chance of having a stroke.[8] That's a pretty good reason to take depression seriously and seek treatment if you have it.

What about if you already have had a stroke? It is beyond doubt that treatment of depression after a stroke is safe and effective. Numerous studies show good results with both older and newer antidepressant medications.[9] My own experience treating depression in stroke patients bears this out. I see stroke patients in my office and in a number of rehab and long-term-care settings, and prescribe antidepressants, psychotherapy, and integrative interventions based on patients' individual needs and preferences (more about this in the chapters of part 3).

Without a doubt, relief from the anguish of depression is a good enough reason to have treatment. But there are other important benefits. Research shows that treatment with antidepressant medications enhances neurological recovery after a stroke and improves functioning and cognitive ability in those with post-stroke depression. To understand how treatment with antidepressant medications helps the brain heal and eventually function better, we turn again to BDNF.

Recall that selective serotonin reuptake inhibitor antidepressants (or SSRIs, and maybe certain other antidepressants) increase BDNF activity in the brain. This promotes neuroplasticity in those recovering from stroke, even in the absence of depression. Some stroke centers now give Prozac or other SSRI antidepressants to their stroke patients, whether or not they are depressed, but this is not yet a universally accepted standard of care.

And, finally, stroke victims treated with antidepressant medications live longer. The amazing thing is that this benefit of antidepressant medications occurs whether or not depression is present.[10]

CONCLUSION

We wrap up this chapter with the lessons learned from Juliette, Sydney A, and Sydney B, the three stroke victims we have met thus far. All three got old before their time as a result of stroke. In each case, depression had a lot to do with it. Juliette might have avoided her stroke had she undergone treatment for depression years earlier. Treatment of post-stroke depression helped Sydney A get back his life back—not 100 percent but close enough. In contrast, untreated depression steered Sydney B down a path of declining health, poor quality of life, and institutionalization. For all intents and purposes, this was a downward spiral of accelerated aging, ultimately leading to premature death, a fate Sydney A avoided. The difference, almost certainly, was treatment of depression.

Doctors routinely counsel their patients about lifestyle modifications to prevent stroke. They prescribe medications for high blood pressure, elevated cholesterol, diabetes, and heart rhythm problems (especially atrial fibrillation), in part, to prevent stroke. Patients' desires to avoid having a stroke are usually so strong that they readily agree to take risky anticoagulant medications. Yet the same doctors do not routinely diagnose or treat depression in their older patients. And the patients who willingly take risky medications to prevent stroke too often deny that depression is a problem or decline treatment for depression if it is offered. This really is too bad because proper diagnosis and treatment of depression clearly prevents a lot of avoidable misery related to stroke.

8

DEPRESSION AND DIABETES

Arnold's daughters, Andrea and Allison, brought him to see me for a second opinion about whether he could continue to live alone. A visiting nurse told them that Arnold had dementia and that he was too confused to live alone safely. The primary care doctor agreed and suggested to Andrea and Allison that they put Arnold in a nursing home, where his diabetes could be managed. They were disheartened, but the writing was on the wall, and, sadly, they began to tour local nursing homes.

Fortunately, the admissions director in one facility had brought her own mother to me a few years earlier, and she recommended that Andrea and Allison hear what I had to say about Arnold before making a final decision. Hoping against hope, they scheduled an appointment for me to evaluate Arnold. In Arnold's case, their hope paid off. I was able to pull him back from the edge of the cliff.

When I met Arnold, he was ninety-two years old. He had been a widower for six years. After his wife died, Arnold continued to live alone in the family home. Arnold had made a decent living as a draftsman and was comfortable in retirement. The house was modest, but it had served his family well and contained many cherished memories. Arnold had no intention of leaving it.

Until this time, Arnold's health had been pretty good. He developed type 2 diabetes about ten years earlier, but he'd been able to control this with diet, exercise, and oral medication. Every day he religiously took a two-mile walk. For two or three years he'd been mildly forgetful.

But this didn't limit him in any way. He paid his bills, balanced his checking account, filed his own tax returns, managed his retirement funds, cooked for himself, and drove. And he took care of his diabetes, including checking his blood sugar, with a draftsman's precision.

Things started to change about one year before I met Arnold. Uncharacteristically he'd started to feel discouraged and negative. He felt he had lived too long, thought that life wasn't so good anymore, and wondered what was the point of going on. Arnold had always been an easygoing individual, with a sunny outlook. Now he was tense, easily upset, negative, and testy. His daughters didn't make too much of this. They assumed it was a normal reaction to old age, widowhood, and loneliness. They tried to get him interested in attending the senior center, but he just scoffed. Diabetes, which had never been more than a minor nuisance to Arnold, now felt like an unbearable hassle that he couldn't bother with. He became lax with his diet, gradually stopped eating on schedule, completely gave up checking his sugars or taking daily walks, and took his medication only when he felt like it.

As time went on, Arnold became more and more forgetful. He became sluggish physically and mentally. His hygiene deteriorated, and he became apathetic, mentally sluggish, and very confused. Arnold's daughters became worried and alerted his primary care doctor. A blood test revealed how badly Arnold's diabetes was out of control, and the doctor arranged for a visiting nurse to make home visits to help Arnold get back on track. After a time, it became obvious that Arnold was too mixed up to handle his diabetes. He failed a memory test the visiting nurse gave him, and the primary care physician diagnosed dementia and concluded that Arnold couldn't care for himself any longer. But Arnold did not have dementia!

Arnold had been swept up in a chain reaction of health problems caused by the interaction of diabetes and depression. Until this time, Arnold had enjoyed excellent mental health. It wasn't aging or loneliness that made him depressed. It was years of diabetes, which had gradually damaged the mood circuits in his brain. Depression made Arnold feel low, and it sapped his energy, motivation, and interest in caring for himself, so that he let his diabetes care slip. The erratic blood sugars affected Arnold's brain, making his depression worse. A vicious cycle ensued. The double whammy of diabetes and depression whittled away at Arnold's cognitive abilities until he appeared to have developed dementia.

How did things get so out of control? First, Arnold didn't recognize the depression in himself. To him it felt like an understandable reaction to putting up with diabetes for ten years. He didn't mention that he felt depressed to either his daughters or his doctor, and nobody thought to ask him. Once he became confused, the situation could no longer be overlooked. Since he'd been forgetful for some time and was now confused, everyone, including his primary care physician, jumped to the conclusion that he had dementia.

WE CAN LEARN A LOT FROM ARNOLD

Does Arnold's story trouble you? It troubles me. Unfortunately, Arnold's story is not unusual. I see patients like Arnold every day.

Frail older adults have healthcare problems that are complicated and complex. Healthcare services tend to be organized to diagnose and treat one disease at a time. But older adults' problems more often arise from the interaction of their various conditions. What's needed is to see the big picture and identify and treat the root causes of problems. In Arnold's case it was depression. But healthcare professionals too often unwittingly treat the end results without recognizing underlying illnesses that set everything in motion. Ever-present assumptions about what is normal in old age, which I described in chapter 1, are part of the problem, as they were for Arnold.

Arnold's story illustrates the tangled relationship between diabetes and depression. Both diabetes and depression are common among older adults, so there is a good chance of having both. Living with two or more diseases is the lot of many older adults. The more conditions you have to deal with, the more complicated life gets. Ask any older adult who has to take fifteen or more pills throughout the day, all at different times, and they will tell you. But with diabetes and depression, it is even more complicated. Diabetes and depression interact: each makes the other worse. Because of this, they must be treated together.

As we saw in Arnold's case, failure to diagnose and treat depression propagated a chain reaction. A new problem arose—confusion—and Arnold was diagnosed as having dementia. Had Arnold's daughters not been on top of his situation, the chain reaction might have kept going, with calamitous results. I've seen it time and time again. Confusion might have led to dehydration followed by delirium and then a fall down the cellar stairs. I'll leave it to your imagination how this usually turns out. I think you can see that a simplistic approach of treating one disease at a time is not sufficient in geriatrics. Especially when diabetes and depression occur together.

DEPRESSION AND DIABETES: OH, WHAT A TANGLED WEB . . .

If you or someone you love has both diabetes and depression, it may not be entirely coincidental. It has been known for a long time that there is a relationship between diabetes and depression. Having depression increases the chance of getting diabetes later in life by 65 percent.[1] Milder depression poses a greater risk, possibly because patients tend to live with it and thus have greater lifetime exposure to depression. Studies show the more years of your life you spend in depression, the more chance you have of getting diabetes and of having more complications of it once you do. And 40 percent of diabetics have clinically significant depression, twice the rate of elders without diabetes. To make matters worse, depression remains undiagnosed and poorly treated in two-thirds of diabetic patients.[2] We saw the nearly tragic results of this in Arnold's case.

Depression and diabetes get tangled up together in older adults like a couple in a bad marriage: each brings out the worst in the other. Depression makes diabetes harder to control and diabetes makes depression harder to treat and more prone to relapses. Elevated blood sugar worsens anxiety and mood, causing both anger and sadness, while low blood sugar results in sadness, worry, and nervousness. When sugar metabolism gets back to normal so does mood. And higher levels of glycohemoglobin, a measure of average blood sugar levels over time, are associated with more severe depression and poorer response to antidepressants.[3] As we will see, diabetes and depression must be treated together. To understand why, we will first review what diabetes is and how it can emotionally impact those who have it.

DIABETES 101

What is diabetes? My patients with diabetes often tell me, "Doc, I have sugar," and they are not far off. Most of us understand that diabetes is a condition of too high blood sugar. Remember the physiologic tightrope we all walk? To stay balanced on the tightrope, our blood sugar level must stay within a fairly narrow range. If it gets too high or too low, we fall off the tightrope. People with diabetes have elevated blood sugar because they do not make enough insulin or their bodies have become insensitive to the actions of insulin. Insulin is a hormone that helps sugar enter the body's cells from the bloodstream. In diabetes, the body does not get the sugar it needs for fuel, and the excess circulating sugar causes chemical damage throughout the body.

Metabolism is the way our body's chemistry keeps us on the tightrope. Diabetes is a metabolic disorder. The importance of this is that depression has significant effects on metabolism. Depression increases the level of the stress hormone cortisol, and cortisol increases blood sugar. This gives you an immediate energy surge in times of stress, which is a good thing, but may cause or worsen diabetes over extended periods. Depression also involves abnormalities of the neurotransmitter serotonin, and serotonin affects sugar metabolism. Depression also causes insulin resistance, but this resolves when depression goes away.

The flip side of the relationship between diabetes and depression may have something to do with the fact that insulin does more than just regulate blood sugar. It has actions in the brain that appear to be important in depression and Alzheimer's disease. Insulin resistance is associated with abnormalities of serotonin chemistry and depression. Prozac, an antidepressant medication, improves insulin sensitivity.[4] Depression creates an inflammatory state in the body, and insulin has anti-inflammatory actions,[5] another common denominator of depression and diabetes. And diabetic patients with depression who are treated with insulin have greater improvement in depression than those who receive oral diabetic medications.[6]

Diabetes causes a wide range of symptoms when it is not well controlled. These include cold or numb hands and feet, frequent urination, excessive hunger, abnormal thirst, shakiness, blurred vision, lack of energy, and feeling faint, fatigued, sluggish, weak, sleepy, or just plain sick. Tiredness, sluggishness, lack of energy, and feeling lousy can also be symptoms of depression. When diabetes and depression are both present, these overlapping symptoms make it more confusing for patients and doctors. Depression can sometimes masquerade as diabetes, causing the presence of depression to be overlooked. And even when both are known to be present, the overlap of symptoms can make it hard to tell what's causing what.

Persons with diabetes must be very faithful about taking care of themselves if they hope to avoid long-term complications, which can be devastating. Eye complications include cataracts and retinopathy, a serious condition that can result in blindness. Chronic kidney disease, known as nephropathy, makes life that much more difficult for diabetics and can necessitate hemodialysis. Diabetic cardiovascular disease causes coronary artery disease, stroke, vascular dementia, and peripheral vascular disease. Peripheral vascular disease results in poor circulation in the feet and legs, with skin problems, ulcers, gangrene, and eventually amputations of toes, feet, and legs. Diabetic peripheral neuropathy causes numbness; distressing sensations of cold, tingling, or burning; and severe pain. Having depression increases the likelihood of developing any of these complications of diabetes. Depression also increases the chance of developing diabetic foot ulcers. Severe depression triples the rate of foot ulcers.[7]

And death. Patients with both diabetes and depression together have a higher death rate than do similar patients with diabetes alone. This effect is more pronounced the older you are, so it is especially worrisome for the elderly.[8]

Depression clearly ages diabetic patients well before their time. Fortunately, if diabetic patients are meticulous and conscientious in taking care of themselves, these very serious complications can often be avoided. But it requires day-in-day-out attention and puts a weight of responsibility on patients with diabetes. Responsible adults handle this pretty well, as did Arnold until he got depressed. Depression robs diabetic patients of the determination they need to keep taking good care of themselves.

DIABETES CARE: WHAT DOES IT TAKE?

The practical challenges of living with diabetes demand more effort from people than do most other medical conditions for affected individuals.[9] This is more so for the elderly who may have other health problems to attend to and may take many other medications in addition to those for their diabetes. Cognitive impairment, functional limitations, and social isolation, when present, all increase the challenge further.

It takes a lot to manage diabetes. Much more is involved than simply taking a pill or giving yourself an insulin shot. The routine requires daily attention to how you feel; checking blood sugars, taking pills, or giving yourself a shot; paying attention to what you eat and when you eat; and getting regular exercise. If you smoke, you have to quit, and losing weight helps. Smoking and being overweight make diabetics more resistant to insulin. And if you don't feel well, you have to call your doctor right away; you can't afford to wait to see if it goes away. The daily routine can feel regimented and burdensome. Some patients understandably feel sorry for themselves.

If depression sets in, it may sap patients' resolve to take care of themselves and stick to their care plan, and leave them feeling they can't be bothered with the rigmarole.[10] This is exactly what happened to Arnold. Patients with depression are three times more likely than those without depression not to faithfully carry out their diabetes care. They have a difficult time eating correctly, are prone to gain or lose large amounts of weight, and fail to take their diabetes medications as prescribed. In contrast, diabetic patients who are not depressed generally are more conscientious about monitoring their blood sugar and taking extra medication, when needed, and they tend to be more motivated to exercise. The lapse in diabetes care makes depression worse, and the vicious cycle is then set in motion.

TREATMENT OF DEPRESSION IMPROVES DIABETES

Just as depression interferes with an individual's ability to perform diabetes care, successful treatment of depression restores this ability.

Effective treatment of depression does more that just helping diabetics regain their motivation to take good care of themselves; it also directly improves metabolism, so diabetes is easier to control. Alleviation of depression directly improves physiologic regulation of blood sugar. Fasting blood sugar and glycohemoglobin levels can improve as a result of treatment.

Despite the impact of diabetes, those with depression can still respond to both antidepressant medications and psychotherapy. One study demonstrated good results with a particular form of psychotherapy called cognitive behavioral therapy. In this study, cognitive behavioral therapy worked better than medication, lowering glycohemoglobin levels as much as did medication but producing a longer-lasting benefit.[11]

Regardless of how it works, treatment of depression helps diabetics enormously. The clearest evidence of this benefit has been from a study that demonstrated that treating depression cut the death rate, from *all* causes, in half, over a five-year period.[12]

Treatment of depression needs to be rigorous and definitive. Studies show depression is a recurring illness in diabetics, with episodes returning almost yearly. Treatment must be relentless. Halfway better is not good enough. Patients must achieve remission, which means they feel back to normal. This is the best way to prevent the downward spiral of depression and diabetes.

When antidepressant medications are used, certain differences among them may be important for diabetic patients. The tricyclic antidepressants and mirtazapine may not be ideal choices. They tend to promote weight gain, which makes diabetes harder to control. And diabetics may be more sensitive to the lightheadedness these medications occasionally cause. For many patients with diabetes, the selective serotonin reuptake inhibitor (SSRI) antidepressants, serotonin norepinephrine reuptake inhibitor (SNRI) antidepressants, and bupropion are better choices. They are usually better tolerated by diabetic patients and less likely to promote weight gain. Bupropion may actually cause weight loss.[13] These are just rules of thumb, and treatment must always be individualized. The bottom line is that for any individual the best medication is the one that works.

A HAPPY ENDING FOR ARNOLD

The visiting nurse and primary care doctor had one thing right: it wasn't safe for Arnold to be home alone—not until he got better.

It took some doing, but I convinced Arnold to be hospitalized in a geriatric medical-psychiatry unit of a hospital. In that specialized setting he was able to get integrated treatment for his depression and his diabetes. After two weeks in the hospital, he had improved a lot, but he needed more time to recover his faculties and went to a rehabilitation program in a nursing home for another five weeks. Happily, he then went home and resumed nearly all of his prior routine. It had been a long road back, and it took another four months before his daughters were confident enough in his abilities to let him drive again. In addition to his medication for diabetes, Arnold also had to take two additional pills for depression. He didn't like this but saw it as a small price to pay to get his life back.

CONCLUSION: TAKE CHARGE OF YOUR DIABETES

Diabetes is a chronic disease. For older adults, depression is usually chronic too. Neither condition is simple. Together they spell double trouble. The health of those with both diabetes and depression deteriorates faster. They feel worse, have poorer quality of life, develop more diabetic complications, and die earlier. They truly grow old before their time.

Living better with depression and diabetes means recognizing that they are intertwined. Each makes the other worse. You cannot expect one to get better without simultaneously treating the other. Anyone with diabetes who is depressed should make sure they receive the best possible care for depression.

Things Not to Do

- It's common to slide into negative thinking about diabetes;[14] don't assume it's a natural reaction. It might be depression.

Things to Do

- If you begin to feel discouraged about your diabetes, or fed up with it, and feel down, tell your doctor that you think you might be depressed.
- If your doctor doesn't take your concerns about having depression seriously, get a consultation with a geriatric psychiatrist or other mental health professional.
- Remind yourself over and over that depression is not a sign of weakness or personal failure but a brain disease that can occur as a medical complication of your diabetes.
- The American Diabetes Association recommends that healthcare professionals screen their diabetic patients for depression.[15] Take this to heart; be on guard for depression in yourself, and tell family members to keep an eye on you as well. They'll know right away when you are not yourself. Make sure they know that depression is not a normal reaction to being old or having diabetes but a serious medical illness.

9

BREATHE EASIER

Depression and Chronic Lung Disease

It's the worst feeling ever. That's what patients say about difficulty breathing. Unless you have a lung disease, you probably take breathing for granted. Patients with chronic lung disease don't.

In this chapter we will focus on a form of chronic lung disease called chronic obstructive pulmonary disease, COPD for short. "Pulmonary" means related to the lungs. Emphysema, chronic bronchitis, and chronic asthma are the respiratory diseases that make up this group.

I treat many older adults with COPD. Mostly they come to me for depression. Many have a fair amount of anxiety as well.

My patients with COPD struggle mightily, and I feel for them. They come to my office toting, dragging, or wheeling portable oxygen machines. When I make house calls, I see them tethered to their oxygen machines, which usually sit on the living room floor. The breathing tube that connects the machine to patients' noses gives about a thirty-foot payout in which they can walk around their home. This always reminds me of dogs leashed to a spike in their owners' backyards—except that dogs would run wild if they could. COPD patients have nowhere to go because they get terribly winded after just a few steps.

I've noticed that my patients with COPD often sit in front of big fans blowing right on them. They say this helps them breathe better by supplying more air. But the problem, obviously, is not lack of air in the room; it's that patients can't get the air around them into their lungs.

Feeling air blow on them seems to ease these patients' insecurity about breathing. In a similar vein, in hospitals or nursing homes, patients get upset when I try to close the door for privacy. They'd rather let the whole world hear their problems than do anything that might cut off the supply of air. I have had a few patients who felt so strongly about this that they would not even let me pull the curtain between the hospital beds.

It is pitiful to watch patients with severe COPD labor with every breath. It's as if they are prisoners of war on a forced death march struggling with each step to take the next one. They are totally consumed by the fight to breathe and often can't pay attention to much of what you are saying. This is gut-wrenching to see.

Those who have not yet become this severe often voice regrets about having been smokers. They kick themselves: "If only I'd known then what I know now!" they lament. Some wish they could convince teenagers not to take up smoking, or to quit while there is still time. Guilt and self-reproach are written all over them. They wished they'd heeded the warnings about the harm of smoking. I wish more of those with depression had heeded their doctors' advice to be treated for it. Sam is a case in point.

Sam was seventy-two years old when I met him near the end of his life. He'd started smoking at age seventeen, while he was in the navy. During his tour, Sam became an excellent welder. After a full tour of duty and an honorable discharge, he carried this trade into civilian life and never lacked for good work at a decent wage.

Sam also continued to smoke, the other thing he picked up in the navy. He was a steady worker and smoker, about a pack a day for fifty years. Once the public warnings started about the harmful effects of smoking, Sam's wife, Gladys, tried to get him to quit. He never did. Sam liked to smoke and didn't like being told what to do. He was mostly a nice guy, but he also had a my-way-or-the-highway attitude that could make things difficult. Gladys could usually work around this, but not when it came to smoking.

Trouble started after Sam turned sixty. He was used to lugging around heavy equipment but now became winded easily. Then came the cough that wouldn't go away. After much procrastination on Sam's part, Gladys finally got him to go to the doctor. His chest x-ray and breathing tests told the story: Sam had emphysema. Prescription inhalers helped, and Sam was able to continue working. He was supposed to exercise, but he rationalized that he got enough exercise at work. And he needed to quit smoking, but he didn't.

Gradually Sam's breathing worsened, and he had to retire at sixty-three. He had nothing to do but sit around the house smoking. Boredom set in quickly and, on its heels, depression. This began with a negative, pessimistic attitude. He felt down in the dumps and felt more and more useless and good for nothing. He started to dwell on his breathing and became consumed with worry about what emphysema would do to him. Every morning he woke at four o'clock and lay awake with negative thoughts racing through his mind. He began to wonder whether he'd be better off dead, but this former sailor was not the type to surrender.

Gladys urged Sam to talk to his doctor about how depressed he'd become, but Sam would have no part of it. He wasn't crazy; his problem was breathing. Was he supposed to be happy about it? No, depression was expectable and normal under the circumstances. Gladys spoke to the doctor anyway, and he wrote a prescription for the antidepressant sertraline (Zoloft), but Sam wouldn't take it.

The former navy welder steamed on, so to speak, but his "boat" was taking on water and eventually it began to sink. One winter he was hospitalized twice with pneumonia. After the first episode he came home with nebulizer treatments. A nebulizer is a machine that aerosolizes inhaled medication into a mist that can be inhaled deeper into the lungs. After the second episode, Sam was discharged from the hospital on home oxygen. He remained weak and discouraged. The cough was constant, and breathing was a struggle. Sam became more deeply depressed and more severely anxious. Anxiety escalated to the point of terror. What would happen when he could no longer breathe?

I met Sam in a rehabilitation hospital. He'd come there to recover after being hospitalized for the fourth time in two years for pneumonia. He weighed only 120 pounds. At his navy "fighting weight," he'd been a strapping five foot ten inches and 172 pounds. He wasn't doing any fighting now, except to breathe. And he was fighting with his physical therapists. He refused all their efforts to convince him to do physical therapy. Sam was afraid that physical therapy would make him more short of breath, and he would never recover from this. He also felt hopeless and saw therapy as futile. He was certain that his doctors had given up on him; he felt he was going to die any time and that the doctors were just going through the motions for his wife's sake.

Sam's doctors believed that his distress was more emotional than respiratory in nature, so they asked me to do what I could to help. When I went to see Sam, he was anxiously calling the nurses every five minutes for help with one thing or another. First it was suctioning the mucus from his upper airway. Next he wanted another nebulizer treatment, even though he knew he couldn't have them more often than every four hours. Finally he needed help to move his fan or adjust his bed, both of which he could do himself. He wore an oxygen mask on his face and had the wide-eyed, terrified stare of a deer in headlights.

The man I met was a shell of himself, a living ghost. He was so on edge that when I entered the room he nearly jumped out of bed in alarm. There was a twenty-four-inch fan on his bedside table not three feet from him, blowing air on him full blast. Before I could introduce myself, he screamed at me not to close the door, for fear it would cut off the air supply. Doing this left him coughing and gasping for air.

Once he regained his composure, or what was left of it, Sam agreed to talk to me. He looked as if he felt that every question I asked him would be the one to finish him off. He wasn't far off base. Every breath he took seemed to me like a do-or-die effort. Speaking left him more winded, and he had to rest between each answer. He was able to speak to me for only five minutes.

I couldn't tell what frightened Sam more, dying or not being able to breathe. Clearly he had little time left—days, weeks, or maybe a month or two. There was not much I could do for him except help to make him more comfortable. I recommended medications to ease his anxiety without further weakening his breathing or making him confused. But I was really too late. Sam had needed me five or six years earlier, when I might have helped him with depression. Had I been able to convince him to accept treatment and relieved his depression, I might then have also been able to help him quit smoking. He might have died of emphysema eventually anyway but not this way and not for at least several more years.

WHAT IS COPD?

By now I'm sure you have a pretty clear picture that COPD is a family of utterly miserable breathing disorders that typically affect people later in life. These illnesses cause difficulty breathing by interfering with airflow deep in the lungs. As I mentioned before, emphysema, chronic bronchitis, and chronic asthma are three major forms of COPD. Many patients have features of both emphysema and chronic bronchitis, and they are referred to as having COPD.

COPD currently is the third leading cause of death in the United States, where it affects fifteen million people.[1] Eighty percent of all cases of COPD are caused by smoking.[2] For those who smoke, the most important aspect of treatment is smoking cessation. Avoiding tobacco smoke and removing other air pollutants from the patient's home or workplace are also important.

Unfortunately, nicotine is highly addictive, and quitting smoking is not so easy. Any smoker will tell you this. Depression makes quitting much more difficult. I usually recommend to my patients who smoke that we deal with their depression first and worry about their smoking once they feel well enough to take this on.

Shortness of breath is usually the first sign of COPD. Patients get winded doing routine tasks such as walking the dog or carrying groceries from the car. Other common symptoms include wheezing, coughing, tightness in the chest, and heavy mucus production. A congested cough first thing in the morning is common. Tiredness, fatigue, and lack of energy are also part of the picture.

Early in the course of COPD, the symptoms can be relieved with medications, mostly inhalers. These help many patients maintain fairly active lives. But COPD is progressive. As the condition worsens, sufferers gradually deteriorate. Respiratory infections are frequent and severe. Hospitalization is often necessary, and during these episodes patients may require help breathing from mechanical ventilators. Even during relatively well periods, breathing may be labored. Weight loss occurs, the lips and fingernails appear bluish, and frailty sets in.

As COPD worsens, quality of life becomes poor. Little activity is possible. Pulmonary rehabilitation may help. This is an individualized treatment program that teaches COPD management strategies to improve quality of life. This may include breathing strategies, energy-conserving techniques, and nutritional counseling. Nebulizers may be needed to relieve severe shortness of breath. Patients who have low blood oxygen levels are often given supplemental oxygen.

If depression has not already been present for some time, it often appears now. Anguish, worry, despair, fear, and hopelessness become part of patients' daily experience. Panic attacks are common. Take my word for it, severe COPD is not a pleasant picture. But it doesn't have to be this bad. Treatment of depression, when present, can avoid much of the suffering associated with COPD.

COPD IS DEPRESSING

Having COPD increases the chance of getting depression by 69 percent.[3] This should come as no surprise to anyone who has chronic lung disease or has known someone with it. In fact depression is very common among persons with COPD. Nearly half of patients with chronic lung disease have some level of depression, and at least one fifth have major depression, the most severe, disabling form of depression.[4]

Living with COPD can be a miserable and very stressful hour-to-hour struggle. Depression drains energy and replaces the fortitude needed to keep going with hopelessness and despair. It makes simple tasks feel insurmountable to healthy individuals; to those with COPD, depression makes everything seem impossible. While it may not be surprising that persons with chronic lung disease get depression, few people appreciate that depression makes chronic lung disease worse.

DEPRESSION WORSENS CHRONIC LUNG DISEASE

When patients with chronic lung disease have depression, they experience greater difficulty breathing. This is not just a subjective experience: depressed patients with COPD perform worse on breathing tests given by respiratory specialists. Daily functioning is poorer than predicted by the breathing disorder alone. Depressed patients cough more and cough up more mucus.[5] Moreover, depression increases the rate of lung disease flare-ups and hospitalizations, and doubles the rate of death over five years.[6]

Part of the impact depression has on COPD is behavioral. COPD patients with depression are much more likely to continue smoking and even increase how much they smoke. Those without depression have more success quitting.[7] And depression makes older adults more sedentary and less inclined to follow prescribed exercise regimens.

THE BRAIN AND RESPIRATORY FUNCTION

Depression has physiologic effects that also worsen COPD. All aspects of breathing and respiratory function are under the control of the nervous system. This connection enables the lungs to respond to circumstances that increase the body's demand for oxygen. But it also provides a route for depression to affect breathing.

The lungs must constantly adjust to meet the body's changing demands for oxygen. The brain monitors the body's condition and environmental circumstances all the time. Through the nervous system, it stays in close communication with all the organs, including the lungs. The lungs have a rich supply of nerves, which allows the brain to adjust breathing rapidly. Signals from the brain can narrow or widen the caliber of airways in the lungs.

Acute stress causes the airways to open up more. This makes passage of air in and out of the lungs easier in times of crisis, when demand is high. If you have to run to escape danger, then your heart has to pump faster and your lungs have to exchange more air, both at a second's notice. This is great in emergencies.

Problems arise under conditions of chronic stress or depression. During episodes of clinical depression, the stress hormones norepinephrine and cortisol are elevated for prolonged periods. This may eventually cause the airways to narrow. Nerve signals coming from the brain during depression may also cause the airways to narrow. This effect is not noticeable to those with healthy lungs but can make breathing much more difficult for those with chronic lung disease. Depression also triggers an inflammatory response throughout the body. In the lungs this narrows the airways and increases secretion of mucus.[8]

TREATMENT OF DEPRESSION IMPROVES LUNG FUNCTION IN CHRONIC LUNG DISEASE

Just as depression makes respiratory function worse in chronic lung disease, treatment of depression can improve it. The benefits include reduced air hunger, anxiety, and fear; improved day-to-day function; and fewer respiratory relapses. Treatment of depression also reduces disability associated with difficulty breathing and improves blood oxygenation and lung airflow.[9]

Treatment of depression lessens the chance of dying with COPD. Chronic lung disease patients who receive treatment for their depression have about half the rate of death over a two-year period.[10] But they have to stick with the treatment. Older adults with COPD more often than not object to treatment with antidepressants.[11] Such objections are very common in my experience, but I have found that with time and patience most patients' reservations can be resolved to their satisfaction. Mental health specialists' skills are often needed to deal with patients' unjustified negative attitudes. The reluctance many older adults have about taking antidepressant medications is such an important problem that I will address it in two separate chapters in part 3.

The good news is that we know antidepressant medications are effective for depression in patients with COPD. Even better news is that pulmonary rehabilitation sometimes relieves depression just as well.[12] So if patients have enough ambition for rehabilitation, it may be worth trying this first. Antidepressants can be reserved for those who do not get better or are too depressed to attempt rehabilitation.

The effectiveness of pulmonary rehabilitation in treating depression illustrates an important principle of treatment of older adults with depression, which applies to other health problems: if rehabilitation programs bring about improvement in physical functioning that patients can see, their outlook may improve and depression may lift. Whether it be stroke rehab, cardiac rehab, orthopedic rehab, or pulmonary rehab, it might be reasonable to put antidepressant treatment on hold to see how much emotional progress they make in rehab.

ZYBAN FOR SMOKING CESSATION

This is not a book on smoking cessation, but we are on the subject and I feel I must mention the role of one antidepressant, bupropion (brand name Zyban), for smoking cessation. A wide range of antidepressant medications may be suitable for many patients with COPD, but bupropion specifically helps patients quit smoking. Smokers do not have to have depression to benefit from bupropion. Bupropion is not a selective serotonin reuptake inhibitor (SSRI) or a serotonin norepinephrine reuptake inhibitor (SNRI), two types of antidepressants I have discussed in prior chapters. It is in a class by itself.

The majority of older adults tolerate bupropion well and have no side effects from it at all. Bupropion can cause trouble sleeping if taken too late in the day. And some patients will get loose bowels, nausea, or jitters. Weight loss is another possibility. Bupropion also increases the chance of having a seizure in those patients at heightened risk for seizures.

A POSTMORTEM FOR SAM

I never saw Sam again. He went home with home hospice care. I provided some telephone advice to the hospice team about ways to keep him comfortable. Then the calls stopped until Gladys called to tell me that Sam had died and to thank me for my help. After that, I never heard from her again.

I mention Gladys at the end of this chapter because I have treated many cases of bereavement depression among widows and widowers of deceased smokers who died of COPD. Some of these mourners experience complicated, mixed feelings about the deceased, and they become depressed. They are terribly sad and bereft yet at the same time feel resentment toward their dead spouse and tremendous guilt over this.

As Gladys did, these spouses provided unwavering care to their mates, watching them dwindle away, gasping for breath . . . and all the while continuing to smoke! I have witnessed the loving devotion of these husbands and wives. While their loved one was still with them, they never faltered. But afterward, they wrestled emotionally with anger and bitterness about their spouses' failure to quit smoking and, in cases such as Sam's, to accept treatment for depression. Most people know about secondhand smoke, but this is "secondhand anguish," and it is a terrible legacy for depressed smokers with COPD to leave behind.

10

DEPRESSION AND CHRONIC KIDNEY DISEASE

One of the many normal, expectable changes associated with aging is a slow, gradual decline of kidney function. This has little significance for the vast majority of older adults. It just means that eighty-year-old kidneys are not as efficient as forty-year-old kidneys. But most old kidneys still get the job done well enough to keep their owners healthy.

Chronic kidney disease (CKD) is a group of illnesses that cause unhealthy loss of kidney function. There are five stages of CKD, from stage 1, the mildest, to stage 5, the most severe. The kidney damage in CKD is permanent, but treatment can slow or prevent further decline. I see many older adults with stage 3 CKD. Those who take good care of themselves usually avoid serious problems. Patients with stage 4 CKD often feel sick. Stage 4 is ominous because it is the last stop before stage 5, complete kidney failure. Complete kidney failure means that the kidneys have given up the ghost, and either a kidney transplant or dialysis is needed to go on living. CKD represents a type of accelerated aging, and depression makes it worse.

Personally, I find the kidneys quite interesting, but unless you have CKD, or someone you care about has it, you have probably not given much thought to your kidneys. You have two of them, kidneys, that is. Each is about the size of your fist, and they sit under the muscles in your flanks, one on each side. The kidneys' main job is to make urine by filtering excess water and waste from the bloodstream. They also maintain electrolyte balance, regulate blood pressure, and make hormones involved in blood pressure control, red blood cell production, and bone health. In CKD the kidneys do not perform these functions adequately. Wastes build up in the bloodstream, fluid and electrolyte imbalances occur, and anemia, osteoporosis, and blood pressure problems crop up.

CKD is a fairly common disorder. It affects 13 percent of the population[1] but is mostly a disease of middle age and older adulthood. Diabetes and high blood pressure are the two major causes of CKD. Together, these diseases account for the vast majority of CKD among older adults. When either of these two conditions is present, proper care of patients with CKD depends on excellent control of them as well. This makes CKD an exceptionally complicated disease, especially for those who also have depression.

Most of the time CKD starts gradually, and the symptoms are fairly general. The symptoms of CKD include tiredness, lack of energy, trouble concentrating, poor appetite, sleep disturbance, swollen feet and ankles, puffiness around the eyes, frequent urination, and dry, itchy skin. You may have noticed that some of the symptoms of CKD are also symptoms of depression. This overlap can make depression difficult to recognize among CKD patients[2] and is probably one reason eight out of ten patients who have CKD and depression do not receive treatment for depression.[3]

Chronic kidney disease places many demands on patients. Patients with CKD must pay constant attention to how they feel. They must keep track of the sodium, potassium, and protein contents of food, and always think about what to eat, how much to drink, and when to take pills. Nothing can be taken for granted, which means that patients with CKD are never fully free of it. In this way CKD shares much in common with diabetes; those with both disorders face a lifestyle double whammy.

Then there are all the doctor visits. In addition to regular visits with primary care physicians and kidney specialists (the latter are called nephrologists), there may be additional appointments with cardiologists or diabetes specialists . . . and maybe psychiatrists, too. My patients often complain, "That's all I do is go to doctors!" Usually they are quick to reassure me that they don't mind coming to see me.

In my experience, the possibility of having to go on dialysis looms constant in the minds of most patients. The vigil over the numbers adds to the stress. "What numbers?" you ask. The numbers are blood tests for sodium, potassium, phosphorus, protein, blood urea nitrogen (BUN), creatinine, creatinine clearance, and glomerular filtration rate (GFR). These lab values measure various aspects of kidney function, among other things. Taken together, they tell nephrologists how the kidneys are doing and help them know how to adjust treatment. They also indicate when complete kidney failure occurs and dialysis must begin.

Unless they have Alzheimer's disease also, my patients with depression usually know what their latest numbers are. When I ask them how they feel, their answers often revolve around "the numbers" and what their nephrologist said about them. I notice that when the numbers are worse, they feel more depressed. Those in stage 4 CKD usually know the exact number at which they will have to start dialysis. They dread each trip to the doctor to review their latest blood work.

As long as they remain free of depression, the majority of patients with CKD handle all this fairly well. Even those on dialysis usually manage to take it in stride. Sure, they complain that dialysis is inconvenient and time consuming. Some find it boring, and others feel drained after each session. Most say it cramps their style. But absent depression, they carry on without letting CKD become a dark cloud hanging over them.

Depression is a game changer. A spirit of determination gives way to self-pity. Minor inconveniences come to feel like unbearable burdens. Hopefulness is replaced by gloom-and-doom thinking. Those on dialysis sometimes start to think that being kept alive "artificially" is no way to live. Such thoughts may lead to considerations of suicide or withdrawing from dialysis to bring on a natural death.

SYLVIA'S CLOSE CALL

In her fifties Sylvia developed type 2 diabetes and high blood pressure. Sylvia was a Brazilian immigrant who had a made a good life for herself working as a nurse's aide in a nursing home. She prided herself on always taking good care of her patients and often received the employee-of-the-month award. But she didn't take as good care of her own diabetes or high blood pressure, and she paid the price. At age sixty-five, she developed CKD. Fortunately she was in stage 2, and Sylvia heard the wake-up call: she started taking good care of herself, and it paid off. For the next two years Sylvia's kidney function did not get any worse.

Then depression struck. Sylvia's usually sunny disposition turned dour and negative. The future looked gloomy, and suddenly she couldn't see any point to worrying about her health any longer and stopped taking good care of herself. Over time, her kidney functions worsened. She started to worry about having to go on dialysis. Everything seemed hopeless, and dialysis seemed inescapable. Sylvia decided she would rather die than live on dialysis.

Sylvia's nephrologist lectured her about the need to take better care of herself. The doctor reassured Sylvia that dialysis could be avoided. But Sylvia's depression got worse, and she developed a delusion that her doctors were falsifying her numbers in order to force her into dialysis. She saw this as part of a government conspiracy to control and deport Latinos.

The nephrologist recognized the depression but didn't tumble to the delusion. She prescribed a selective serotonin reuptake inhibitor (SSRI) antidepressant, but when it didn't help she referred Sylvia to me.

By the time I met Sylvia, she was sad, morose, sluggish, and withdrawn. She also had periods of confusion. Sylvia told me she didn't want to die, but she didn't want to go on living either if it meant being on dialysis. She had begun to have thoughts about ways to commit suicide. Much of her thinking didn't make sense. I suspected that Sylvia was getting confused from the additive effects of severe depression and the wastes building up in her bloodstream. Fortunately, with her family's encouragement, Sylvia accepted treatment for depression and improved quickly. She resumed taking very good care of herself, and her kidneys gradually improved. Sylvia dodged the dialysis bullet.

DEPRESSION AND CKD

Depression is the most common mental health problem among patients with chronic kidney disease. Among those who do not yet need dialysis, one in five has major depression, but up to half have less severe, but no less significant, clinical depression.[4] Patients on dialysis are even more likely to have depression.[5]

Maybe it seems obvious to you that many patients with CKD have depression. After all, chronic kidney disease is nothing to be happy about. But depression is more than an understandable, normal reaction to CKD. The relationship between depression and CKD is much more complicated. If you have read all the previous chapters, maybe you no longer find this surprising.

Living with CKD is highly stressful, and as we now know, prolonged stress can trigger brain changes that result in depression. The metabolic wastes that accumulate in the blood in CKD have toxic effects on the brain that include depression. And we also know that high blood pressure and diabetes, which often cause CKD, independently cause depression through circulatory changes in the brain.

Depression also makes CKD worse. Older adults with CKD who also develop depression have greater disability, more cognitive impairment, and poorer quality of life.[6] Depression makes patients with CKD more likely to be hospitalized, start dialysis, or die.[7]

HOW DOES DEPRESSION MAKE KIDNEY DISEASE WORSE?

Depression makes chronic kidney disease worse in a number of ways. First, patients who are depressed have a much harder time following their treatment and taking proper care of themselves. This should also seem like a familiar story. Successfully managing life with CKD requires motivation, determination, organization, and planning. It's doable if you are not depressed but very tough if you are. However, patients who do not take good care of themselves don't always have depression. People neglect their health for many reasons. Depression is a common one.

Second, the heightened levels of stress hormones in depression have harmful effects on the kidneys. Cortisol causes sodium retention and increases blood pressure. Over long periods of time, this damages the kidneys further.[8] Depression also increases inflammation and oxidative damage throughout the body, and this can aggravate kidney damage as well.[9]

THE GOOD NEWS

Fortunately, depression can be treated in those with CKD, and treatment improves their quality of life. Psychotherapy, antidepressant medications, and exercise may help.[10] Patients with CKD, including those on dialysis, usually tolerate antidepressant medications well. Many get better, if they take the medications. Unfortunately, many patients with CKD feel sick and tired of taking pills and object to adding antidepressant medications.[11] More on this later.

So, while we know that depression makes CKD worse, and depression in CKD can be treated successfully, it has not yet been proven that treating depression in CKD prevents CKD from getting worse. But not treating it is clearly bad. Patients with CKD mostly die of cardiovascular disease, and treating depression forestalls this fate. Because the impact of depression is so great, and the consequences so dire, experts in kidney disease recommend screening all patients with CKD for depression and treating it.[12]

EASIER SAID THAN DONE

Just because patients with CKD can be successfully treated for depression does not mean it's always easy. First there is the hurdle of patients' objections to get over. Then there are the drugs themselves. Fortunately, the majority of antidepressant medications are metabolized by the liver, which means dialysis patients can take them. Some antidepressants have metabolites that are cleared by the kidneys, and these must be used cautiously to prevent toxic levels from accumulating in the body. In many cases, lower doses must be prescribed. The SSRI antidepressants can be a good choice for patients with CKD as long as extra caution is taken against bleeding or nausea and vomiting.[13]

DEPRESSION AND DECISIONS TO DECLINE OR WITHDRAW FROM DIALYSIS

Dialysis can extend life and improve its quality for many patients with CKD. But some find that it only prolongs a life of misery and delays a dignified, natural death. Patients with such outlooks sometimes decide to decline starting dialysis or, if they already are receiving it, to discontinue it. Obviously this is not a simple medical decision but involves moral, ethical, religious, and family considerations, which are beyond what I can address here (the National Kidney Foundation has a web page that addresses this very nicely).[14] But I do want to talk about the impact of depression on this most profound life-and-death decision.

The right to refuse medical treatment is, under most conditions, sacrosanct in our healthcare system. This right extends to those who refuse life-saving or life-sustaining treatments, including dialysis. But it rests on the presumption that people's decisions are sound and based on their long-held beliefs and values. One issue raised when a patient declines dialysis is whether that decision is sound. Depression can make thinking unduly negative, pessimistic, and hopeless, robbing those severely affected of their ability to make sound decisions.

Sylvia was headed down this path. She considered committing suicide rather than face dialysis and would have likely refused it. Her preference that death was better than life on dialysis was colored by depression and did not represent her true thinking. Once her depression was treated, she had a different attitude.

When someone feels sad about having an awful disease for which there is no cure and no reprieve, others may sympathize with his or her decision not to go on living, seeing it as understandable and natural. They may not recognize depression or its impact on the person's thinking. Patients' family members often question why this matters, and here is what I tell them. If patients with depression receive treatment, and if they get better, they often make different decisions. I have treated many depressed patients who refused life-sustaining treatments, including dialysis, but decided to have those treatments once they responded to treatment. Here's the bottom line: while deciding to stop dialysis and allow a natural death to occur can be the right decision for some patients, no person should die of, or with, depression. Dialysis patients' decisions to withdraw from treatment must be respected, but their doctors and family members should determine if their decision represents their true wishes or is their depression talking. When present, depression should be treated first before final decisions are made about continuing or stopping dialysis.

Most of us do not give much thought most of the time to how we will die. We try not to think about it. In my experience, many older adults with chronic, progressive diseases such as CKD give a lot of thought to how they will die. The majority of those with whom I have worked say that at the end they hope to be alert, sharp, and of clear and sound mind. Depression thwarts this hope, but it doesn't have to. We'll come back to this topic again in the next chapter, on cancer.

CONCLUSION

Earlier, I didn't tell you what it took to get Sylvia well. Before I started treating her, she was already on two diabetes medications, two blood pressure medications, a thyroid pill, medications to reduce cholesterol and stomach acid, a baby aspirin, and the antidepressant medication her nephrologist had prescribed. All told, she had to take ten medications, corresponding to twelve pills per day. To make her better, I recommended switching to a different antidepressant and adding an antipsychotic medication. This increased the number of daily pills to fourteen.

The situation was not promising. Sylvia was adamantly against taking any more pills. On top of this, she was not taking care of herself, and her thinking had become irrational. I worried that she would need to be hospitalized. Fortunately, her family was kind, loving, supportive, and helpful, and they took care of her. I saw her in my office twice a week and worked closely with her family. Together, we were able to convince Sylvia to try additional medication, and family members were terrific in making sure she took them, as well as seeing to her needs.

Sylvia accepted the additional medications and had no difficulty with the antipsychotic medication. It was not so easy with the antidepressant. I decided to skip over the SSRI antidepressants because I was concerned about an increased risk of bleeding related to her kidney disease. I ruled out a few other choices that have metabolites that are cleared by the kidneys. The first drug that I did try quickly increased her blood pressure, so it had to be stopped. Yet another made her nauseated. Naturally, these problems did not make Sylvia any more receptive to medications, but she continued to take them. Such "false starts" in treating geriatric depression are common and are one reason treatment of depression can take a long time. We'll look at this problem in depth in chapter 21. Finally, we found an antidepressant medication that agreed with Sylvia, and she began to get better.

The first sign of improvement was that Sylvia started to take better care of herself. Then she stopped being afraid that her doctors were plotting to put her on dialysis. Little by little she continued to improve, and by the seventh week she seemed mostly back to normal. At four months, Sylvia was handling all her pills without help, following her diet religiously, and exercising at a health club three times a week. She no longer felt despair, had no further reservations about living with CKD, and was determined to do everything possible to keep her disease under control. Most important, she now felt that should she need dialysis it would not be the end of the world. She could live with it.

11

DEPRESSION AND CANCER

My patient Judith once told me, "I've had both depression and cancer. If I had to have either one again, I'd take the cancer. There's nothing as bad as depression." What a choice, depression or cancer! I treated Judith for depression about fifteen years ago, but her statement made a lasting impression on me. Is depression really worse than cancer? People die of both, but some live their entire lives with depression and the same cannot be said about cancer. What I have learned from treating many patients with cancer, who came to me for depression, is that patients with both diseases are truly cursed. Their suffering is hard to watch.

Actually, I don't really care which is worse, depression or cancer. Both are horrible afflictions. The point I hope to leave you with in this chapter is that if you have cancer and depression you need to address both with equal seriousness. Most people dread cancer above all else. Very few dread depression enough. Too many individuals still view depression as an expected, normal reaction to depressing circumstances and something that can be ignored. Cancer patients who ignore depression surrender to cancer without realizing it.

As if anything could make cancer worse, depression actually does in several ways. Perhaps most alarming is that depression can make you more likely to get cancer. Once you have cancer, depression makes it worse. It increases misery, makes the cancer advance faster and come back earlier, and makes you more likely to die from cancer. Given the stakes, it is even more critical that those with cancer who have depression get treatment for their depression. We will look at all these aspects of depression and cancer in this chapter. You will notice many similarities with other diseases covered in earlier chapters.

CANCER IS NOT DEPRESSING . . . REALLY?

What could be more depressing than being told you have cancer? Surprisingly, cancer doesn't make people more likely to get depression, at least not in the sense of the depressive illnesses we covered in chapter 4. The majority of patients with cancer do not get depression. This remains true even among terminal patients. In one study of patients with metastatic lung cancer, who on average had less than one year to live, fewer than one out of six patients had major depressive disorder, and suicidal feelings were rare.[1]

Sure, many cancer patients feel depressed. Who wouldn't? Cancer is a dreaded condition. Receiving the diagnosis, living with the disease, and enduring its treatment can be utterly miserable, full of anguish, fear, and despair. Such feelings are common and normal, but they do not necessarily signify the presence of depressive illness any more than during mourning for the death of a loved one. In the absence of depressive illness, patients with cancer cope with their disease fairly well.

DEPRESSION IS COMMON AND TOO OFTEN IGNORED

Rates of depression in cancer are variable. Some studies show that cancer patients are no more likely to get major depressive disorder than anyone else. Others show as many as half of all patients with cancer also have serious depressive symptoms. Do you find this confusing? That's because researchers study different types of cancer and apply different definitions of depression. You probably do not find it surprising that many cancer patients have depression. Keep in mind that for every cancer patient who has depression, at least one does not, so depression is not inevitable.

What surprises me is how much depression is neglected among cancer patients.[2] Neither patients nor their doctors pay much attention to it. Only 15 percent of patients with cancer and depression receive adequate treatment for depression. I suspect, as I alluded to earlier, that cancer draws everyone's attention, leaving depression lurking in the shadows.

This is not to say that cancer shouldn't command a five-alarm response. It's just that the overwhelming emphasis of cancer research has been on treatment for the cancer itself, and little attention has been paid to depression and other complications.[3] The result is that too many cancer doctors (known as oncologists) are still not tuned in to the need to address depression in their patients, and they are not up to speed in diagnosing and treating depression in their patients.

Part of the problem oncologists face is that depression is harder to recognize in some patients with cancer. As we saw with chronic kidney disease, many of the symptoms of cancer and depression overlap. Fatigue, poor appetite, weight loss, and pain are symptoms of both depression and many types of cancer.[4] Chemotherapy also causes many of the same symptoms, further muddying the waters.[5]

WHAT IS CANCER?

Before we go on, let's review what cancer is to appreciate the toll depression takes on those who have it.

One of the requirements for you to stay healthy is that the trillions and trillions of cells in your body must all know their place and what they are supposed to do. Skin cells must remain skin cells, stay put in the skin, and keep doing the job of skin cells. The same is true of brain cells, white blood cells, and intestinal cells, to name a few of the many types of cells in the body. Instructions written into your DNA give your cells their marching orders.

Ordinarily, nearly all of the cells in your body follow the script exactly. But some do not. Perhaps thousands of times a day, DNA gets damaged by oxidation or toxins, or mutated during cell division. Fortunately, our cells have built-in safeguards. When this happens the DNA damage is usually repaired. If this fails to happen, the abnormal cell may die on its own or be attacked and killed by your immune system. Either way, all's well, and you are none the wiser.

In cancer, all hell breaks out instead. The damaged DNA is not repaired, and the immune system fails to kill the cell containing the damaged DNA. Instead the cell runs amok. The affected cell forgets its identity and job description and becomes a cancer cell instead; it then begins to reproduce uncontrollably. This leads to a tumor, a lump of cancer cells, which keeps on growing. The unrestrained growth of the tumor causes local trouble—the breast lump felt on self-exam, blockage in the intestine, or a shadow on a chest x-ray. As if this isn't bad enough, cancer cells can break off from the tumor and spread to other parts of the body, wreaking havoc. The growth and spread of cancer occurs at the expense of the healthy parts of the body, eventually consuming it and killing the person.

Imagine your body is a forty-story office building. If a fire breaks out in an office trash can, the sprinkler system will go off and douse it, and the fire alarm will summon the fire department to make sure the fire is contained. In cancer, a water main break means the sprinklers do no good and the fire department's hoses are useless. The building burns to the ground.

With trillions and trillions of cells to police, the body's defensive machinery must perform flawlessly for any of us to live our entire lives cancer free. Given what you already know about the hormonal, inflammatory, and oxidative changes caused by depression, I think you can see how depression could be a monkey wrench in the body's cancer seek-and-destroy machinery.

ALPHABETICAL DISORDER: WHEN D COMES BEFORE C

So dreaded is cancer that people cringe at hearing or speaking it; instead, they refer to it as the "c-word." In the ABCs of cancer, when *d* stands for depression sometimes *d* goes before *c*: some people get depression first and cancer some time later. For some, this misfortune may be coincidental, but for others the depression bears on the cancer to come.

Can depression increase your chance of getting cancer? The scary answer, which seems to me to be a compelling reason not to ignore depression, is yes, possibly. Severe depression increases the chance of getting cancer by 62 percent over a five-year period.[6] The impact may be more dramatic over longer periods of time. We do not yet know.

Depression does not cause cancer in the direct way smoking or asbestos exposure causes lung cancer. Depression is a risk factor for cancer. But how does depression increase the risk of cancer? Again, we don't know for sure. But there are several plausible ways, once again coming back to behavior and physiology.

Individuals with depression are more prone to unhealthy lifestyle choices that increase their risk of cancer. Smoking is the most striking example. While smoking rates have been declining in the Western world, 40 to 60 percent of depressed patients in those countries smoke.[7] Consuming alcohol in moderation, keeping your weight down, eating a low-fat diet, and exercise are healthy practices that reduce the risk of cancer. Public health warnings urge us to do these things to reduce our risk of cancer. But it takes determination, planning ahead, and willpower, traits that persons with depression have in short supply. They smoke and drink too much, eat poorly, and do not exercise.[8] We have seen that this increases their risk for other serious health problems. Add cancer to the list.

Then there are the physiological alterations brought about by depression, including elevated cortisol, increased inflammation, and oxidative stress. We will see shortly that these conditions account, in part, for how depression worsens the course of cancer. For now, I think you'll agree that effects of depression make it more difficult to hold cancer in check, if it arises. In fact, depression weakens the immune system's ability to seek out and destroy abnormal cells before they cause cancer.[9] Depression makes it easier for cancer to gain a foothold.

DEPRESSION MAKES CANCER WORSE

What about if you already have cancer? Researchers and cancer specialists widely believe that depression makes cancer worse.[10] This is no surprise really. How could it not? Having cancer is miserable. Having depression at the same time seems akin to rubbing salt in an open wound. In fact, depression worsens quality of life more than does the cancer itself. My former patient Judith certainly felt this way. Depression is the difference between cancer being something you can cope with and something you can't.

When I met Judith, she was battling colon cancer. Her oncologist had referred her to me because of depression. The cancer had spread beyond her colon to local lymph nodes. Judith had undergone surgery to remove the cancerous section of her colon. This left her with a temporary colostomy, which she was not handling well. She found it disgusting and thought strangers on the street would find her repulsive. Judith had already completed half of the necessary rounds of chemotherapy. These treatments left her very fatigued and tired. She experienced no nausea or vomiting but felt she had a sick spirit—gloom and despair were unshakable. Judith had been wondering whether it was worth going through any more. She had no thoughts of killing herself but felt she, and her family, would be better off if she died in her sleep. The guilt she felt over putting her family members through her cancer was made worse by the feeling that she must have brought this on herself somehow and that it was deserved.

Judith had major depressive disorder, and I treated her with antidepressant medication and psychotherapy. She showed signs of improvement within three weeks and felt nearly back to normal, emotionally, at six weeks. The difference was night and day. The chemotherapy now seemed tolerable. Not only that, the colostomy even felt manageable. She was able to focus on completing the chemotherapy and looked forward to having the colostomy reversed. Looking back, she now saw the colon cancer as miserable but viewed the depression as living hell.

Judith illustrates how depression dramatically adds to the misery of cancer. Unfortunately, that's not the whole story. Having depression on top of cancer leads to worse cancer outcomes. Compared with similar cancer patients without depression, those who have it suffer faster tumor growth, more recurrences, and earlier death. Think about that. Some people die unnecessarily of cancer because they are depressed.[11]

"HOW LONG HAVE I GOT, DOC?"

How often do we hear this melodramatic line spoken in the movies? In one form or another it crosses the minds of most everyone diagnosed with cancer, for obvious reasons.

Over eight million people die of cancer per year worldwide.[12] Despite this staggering number, cancer is no longer the death sentence it used to be. I treat many patients in their eighties and nineties who had cancer earlier in life and are still around. Eventually, they'll die of something else at a ripe old age. These folks have a hearty attitude about cancer, seeing it as just rough times they had to live through. They seem to enjoy bragging that so many years later they are "still on this side of the turf." They must get that line from the same old-age playbook. I suspect that one thing that sets these survivors apart is that they didn't have depression earlier in their lives.

Again, cancer victims with depression have a shorter life expectancy than those who do not. This applies to a wide range of cancers, including prostate cancer,[13] pancreatic cancer,[14] metastatic lung cancer,[15] and breast cancer.[16] The more severe the depression, the greater the impact. Major depressive disorder, one of the most severe forms of depression, shortens life expectancy the most.[17]

Making general comments about cancer is difficult because there are many types, and they all present different challenges. Oncologists diagnose cancer not only by type but also by stage. Staging is based on the size of the tumor, whether it has spread locally into lymph nodes or metastasized to distant areas of the body—basically the stage tells you how big the cancer has grown and how far it has spread.

Early-stage cancer is just that. The fire has not spread beyond the office it started in and can still be put out. In late-stage cancer, the fire has engulfed the whole floor and spread to others. At this stage, more often than not, it's only a question of how long before the whole building goes up.

Due to good early detection, breast cancer is often caught in the early stages. Because of this, it is no longer an automatic death sentence. Women with early-stage breast cancer, who have a relatively small tumor and receive adequate treatment, have more than a 75 percent chance of being alive twenty-five years later.[18] But depression increases their death rate by 42 percent over five years.[19] With those kinds of odds, the last thing someone with breast cancer should do is ignore depression.

Lung cancer is not usually detected until the late stages and provides a dramatic comparison with breast cancer. Late-stage lung cancer patients with depression have, on average, about a year to live, or less, but those without depression live twice as long—two years, on average.[20] If you have depression, though, all is not hopeless. One study showed that patients whose depression improved also lived twice as long as those who continued to be depressed. That extra year, if it is free of depression, can mean a lot to cancer victims. The elderly patients I treat often have different, more modest expectations of life. A little more quality time can mean the world to them once they are free of depression. One of the happiest moments for my patient Clarice was realizing she would live to dance at her great-grandson's wedding. For another, it was a granddaughter's graduation from the U.S. Air Force Academy, one of the proudest moments of her life. Most touching was Daisy, who reached one hundred. She got her congratulatory letter from the president of the United States, which she proudly had framed and hung in the foyer of her house for everyone who entered to see.

We all die. Cancer causes some people to die younger than they otherwise might. We can't change this—not yet. But I strongly believe that no one should die with depression if it can be helped. Why let depression spoil the time you have left or make it even shorter?

HOW DOES DEPRESSION WORSEN CANCER?

More than any illness we have covered so far, early diagnosis matters in cancer. The earlier you catch it, the better your chances. A delay in diagnosis means the cancer will be that much further advanced once you start treatment.

Let's ignore, for a moment, the possibility that depression causes cancer. Whether or not it does, depression delays cancer diagnosis. Depression makes people less inclined to bother with routine screening for diseases. For example, women suffering from depression may not do breast self-examination or have recommended mammograms. People with depression tend to overlook and disregard early warning signs of all diseases and procrastinate getting medical attention for them. Cancer doesn't go away. When it is eventually diagnosed, it will be further along and have a worse prognosis.[21]

Survival with cancer also depends on early and complete treatment. Cancer treatment has become much better but is most successful when patients receive the full course. Anything less increases the odds of the cancer spreading or metastasizing and of premature death. Major depression, in particular, is often associated with loss of will to live.[22]

Family members often express worry to me that their relative seems to have given up. Such patients see no point in going through surgery or enduring chemotherapy. In fact, studies show that cancer patients with depression are less likely to have recommended surgery, chemotherapy, and radiation therapy.[23]

Treatment of cancer can be frightening, arduous, and very unpleasant. Depression makes patients less likely to stick with cancer treatment.[24] When patients have depression, they are more sensitive to toxicity from chemotherapy and less able to endure it.[25]

Friends and family can do much to help persons with cancer overcome these obstacles so they can receive the full treatment they need. Unfortunately, delays in diagnosis and reluctance to have, or complete, treatment do not fully explain how depression makes cancer worse. Studies have looked at treatment outcomes among cancer patients who were fully treated. Even when treatment was thorough and complete, those with depression did worse than those without it. Researchers interpret this to mean that depression makes cancer more aggressive. They blame the high levels of cortisol and inflammation from the depression, which weaken the body's ability to withstand cancer.[26]

WHICH OLDER ADULTS SHOULD HAVE CANCER TREATMENT?

Frailty and the presence of other common illnesses of aging, such as congestive heart failure, chronic obstructive pulmonary disease, and chronic kidney disease, make chemotherapy harder for older adults to withstand. Some will nevertheless want treatment. This can be a good decision for many, and many older adults handle cancer treatment quite well.[27] For others, especially those expected to have a very rough time, or those with a limited life expectancy, cancer treatment may not be the best thing for them.

Which older adults ought to have cancer treatment? How do you decide? These are tough questions that must be made on a case-by-case basis, with the help of various members of the medical team. I have been called in many times to help advise patients and their oncologists. One vital lesson from my experience that I will leave you with is the importance of not allowing depression to unduly influence decisions about treatment.

Having a terminal disease can make patients feel that treatment of depression is futile. Keep in mind that depression can make patients pessimistic, hopeless, illogical, and unreasonable. Their judgment may no longer be sound.

I have seen late-stage cancer patients worry about pain. They want to make sure they will not have agonizing pain from their cancer. At the same time, they fear that pain medications will compromise their lucidity near the end. It has always troubled me that many of these patients who so highly value their lucidity are willing to let themselves go on being depressed. They often accept narcotic pain medications knowing that these drugs can cause mental side effects that may leave them "out of it," confused, and not lucid. Yet they decline antidepressant medications. Antidepressant medications are not narcotics and are not mind altering—quite the opposite. Antidepressants help depressed patients to be mentally sharper and to feel like themselves again. They are mind restoring!

As I said before, no one should die with depression, if they can avoid it, and no one should make decisions to forgo cancer treatment while influenced by depression—at least not without input from a psychiatrist familiar with these matters.

TREATMENT OF DEPRESSION AND CANCER PROGNOSIS

At this point, you might very well ask, "Does treating depression matter in cancer?" Does depression in cancer patients get better? Does this improve the course of cancer? Unfortunately, we do not know. There have been very few studies with either antidepressant medications or psychotherapy, and the results have been mixed.

Despite the lack of proof that treatment of depression makes a difference in cancer, you should still have it if you are depressed. To quote the scientist Carl Sagan, of the original television series *Cosmos*, "Absence of evidence is not evidence of absence." Lack of proof that something exists does not prove that it does not. Research on cancer patients with depression is difficult to do, and the few studies that have been done have weaknesses.

Don't be discouraged about treatment. Why not? First, I have treated depression in many patients with cancer. I have seen a lot of those with early-stage cancer get better. Relief from depression changes their outlook for the better and makes cancer something they feel they can cope with. I have also treated many late-stage or terminal patients. These situations certainly are sadder, and their predicament is more hopeless. Sometimes their depression gets better, other times not. But when depression does get better, the difference in quality of life is enormous.

One thing is clear: successful treatment of depression requires sustained attention from the doctor. As we saw in chronic kidney disease, it is not enough just to prescribe antidepressant medication, because cancer patients are likely to reject it or give up on it too easily. It takes time to make sure patients understand the importance of the treatment and how it will help. Several appointments may be needed, during which the doctor should mostly listen to the patient's concerns and address them as supportively as possible. Patience is needed. If the doctor gives up too easily, you can't expect the patient to avoid doing so as well, since he or she is already in a giving-up mode of thinking. Helping patients overcome this mode of thinking takes time and may require psychological skills.

A SPECIAL CAUTION ABOUT TAMOXIFEN

Many antidepressant medications are suitable for treatment of patients with cancer. One exception applies to breast cancer patients receiving tamoxifen. Tamoxifen is a medication in tablet form given to women with early-stage breast cancer to prevent it from coming back. Breast cancer survivors on tamoxifen who have depression should receive treatment for their depression. But caution is needed. Many antidepressants, including all of the selective serotonin reuptake inhibitors (SSRIs), as well as some others, interfere with tamoxifen's activity, leaving patients more vulnerable to cancer recurrence.[28] Patients taking tamoxifen should avoid these antidepressants.

The good news is that there are many other antidepressants that do not interact with tamoxifen and are safe for breast cancer survivors. Oncologists who treat many breast cancer patients are usually familiar with one or two of these alternatives. If these medications do not work out, consultation with a psychiatrist knowledgeable about treating breast cancer survivors for depression is a good idea.

WHAT CAN FAMILY MEMBERS DO?

Family members and close friends can make a big difference in the life of someone with cancer. Quite literally they may have a life-and-death impact.

Cancer treatment can be overwhelming and confusing. Even the most conscientious patients need help navigating treatment. Essentially, family members are the wingmen, making sure that treatment, including for depression, does not "fall through the cracks."

In addition to providing emotional support, encouragement, and reassurance, family members must be on guard for depression in their loved ones. They must recognize when it has appeared and has made their loved ones unduly pessimistic and inclined to turn down cancer treatment that other patients with the same cancer accept. Cancer is nothing to mess around with. Anything that worsens the odds needs to be addressed urgently. Cancer patients with depression have difficulty advocating for treatment of their depression. Family and friends must do it for them.

12

DEPRESSION AND ARTHRITIS

Daniel was a seventy-six-year-old man still in fairly good health. He had been a police captain in a small city, where he still lived with his wife. They had been happily married for forty-nine years. Daniel was well known around town, and people liked him. After retiring at age sixty-five, Daniel did part-time security consulting, but that dried up after a year or so. Then he had little to do.

Initially, Daniel didn't take to retirement well. He missed the prestige, authority, and sense of accomplishment he got from his law enforcement career. He no longer felt important. Little by little he got used to it. Golf, yard work, and long-neglected household projects, such as painting, kept him reasonably busy.

Winters were tough. There was nothing to do, and he suffered from cabin fever. Snowstorms provided some relief. Nearly all the older patients I treat hate the snow, but Daniel welcomed a good storm. Clearing snow and ice gave him something to do, and he gladly plowed his neighbors' sidewalks and driveways with his snow blower, taking on an informal role as the local snow captain.

Daniel got by this way for a few years until, without fanfare, osteoarthritis arrived and gradually changed things for the worse. First there were the twinges of pain on the golf course, in the shoulders while swinging the club and in the knees and hips while walking the course. Pain then made it all but impossible to mow the lawn, rake leaves, or prune shrubs. Over-the-counter arthritis medications helped a little, but gradually the symptoms worsened.

Daniel went to see his primary care physician, who told him the aches and pains were old-age osteoarthritis. The doctor prescribed a prescription-strength arthritis medication and advised Daniel to slow down and take it easy, but Daniel had no intention of cutting back.

Daniel's body had other ideas. When fall arrived he couldn't play golf, and when winter set in he wasn't able to shovel snow. Daniel sat helplessly inside while his son plowed the driveway and shoveled the walk. As the winter passed, family members noticed Daniel becoming grumpy, negative, and pessimistic. He'd also begun taking naps, something he'd never done before.

Nobody made very much of this change in Daniel's behavior or attitude, attributing both to old age and a bad winter. But things worsened with the coming of spring. Daniel's joint pain and stiffness had increased, he couldn't move his shoulders much, and he'd lost fifteen pounds. By the time golf season opened, Daniel had become too weak and feeble to play. He made no attempt at yard work and did nothing but sit on his porch and stare at his lawn or take long naps.

At this point, Daniel's primary care physician referred him to Dr. Irving, a rheumatologist. Rheumatologists are specialists in joint and connective tissue diseases, and they handle arthritis. Dr. Irving confirmed the diagnosis of osteoarthritis and recommended a treatment plan consisting of a different prescription arthritis medication, physical therapy, and regular exercise. Daniel attended most of the scheduled physical therapy sessions but made no effort to exercise or do his therapy at home.

Daniel's wife became increasingly worried about him. She also felt frustrated with his sitting around the house doing nothing. She began asking him to help her with the housework, but he said he was too sore to push a vacuum cleaner or carry laundry baskets up and down the cellar stairs. Daniel felt more and more discouraged, down in the dumps, and useless. He became more withdrawn and lost interest in doing anything, even sedentary activities.

The rheumatologist also felt frustrated. By all objective indications, Daniel's arthritis was too mild to explain his level of disability. He suspected Daniel might be depressed and referred him to me for an evaluation.

Having heard Daniel's tale, many readers might conclude, "Of course he's depressed. His body has let him down, and he feels useless."

Maybe you are thinking the same thing. I might agree with you except that Daniel is more than "bummed out" over a disabling condition, and arthritis was not what disabled him; depression was.

Remember the difference between feeling down in response to unhappy developments in life, and depressive illness? The former comes and goes in waves, can be shaken off, and does not interfere with normal, day-to-day functioning or cause loss of interest in life. Daniel had a severe form of depressive illness called major depressive disorder. Arthritis caused some of his disability, but depression caused far more.

Over the years, I have treated many patients like Daniel, suffering from both arthritis and depression. Depression and arthritis are both common among older adults and often occur together. In fact, arthritis sufferers have two to three times as much depression as others their age without arthritis.[1]

ARTHRITIS

Arthritis is an inflammatory condition of the joints. Its main symptoms are pain and stiffness, which can restrict mobility, flexibility, and activity. Joint damage eventually leads to visible deformity.

Some degree of arthritis affects more than half of persons over the age of sixty-five and more than 80 percent of those over age seventy-five.[2] Osteoarthritis is the most common form of arthritis affecting older adults, and it is the type Daniel had. Rheumatoid arthritis usually starts earlier in life but also affects older adults.

Unchecked, arthritis causes disability. No surprise there. But arthritis sufferers who also are depressed have more pain, greater limitation of activity, and more disability than similar arthritis sufferers without depression. Depression makes arthritis worse!

DANIEL'S EVALUATION

When I met Daniel he felt blue and gloomy all the time and couldn't snap himself out of it. He was slow moving, achy, sluggish, and weak, and his sleep and appetite were poor. His self-esteem was "in the toilet," and he had no interest or motivation for anything. I thought Daniel was resigned and had given up. He told me he was "all washed up" and "broken down" and there was nothing doctors could do about it, because it was "just old age."

How did arthritis waylay Daniel so quickly? Depression snuck in the back door, undetected by family members, who blamed the arthritis for his deterioration. In my experience, this often happens to older adults with arthritis. People expect arthritis to get worse as time goes by. So when it does, they do not consider the possibility that something else, such as depression, might also be at work.

This pattern, called misattribution, occurs with many progressive diseases.[3] It's an important idea, so I'll restate what it is. When a disease that is known to get worse does, people naturally assume the decline is due to the disease. They fail to consider that something else might be wrong, and so do not recognize the contribution to the symptoms that a second illness is making. The trick is to recognize when the first disease has worsened faster than expected and then look for a reason. This takes some medical expertise. But patients and family members can sound the alert whenever things go downhill faster than expected.

It is easy to miss depression because its symptoms overlap with those of arthritis. Fatigue, loss of appetite, poor sleep, lack of energy, and weight loss are seen in both. While pain is the main symptom of arthritis, depression also causes aches and pains. And both arthritis and depression impair function. We have already encountered this problem as it applied to chronic kidney disease and cancer. Without a red flag to signal the presence of depression, even doctors can mistakenly assume diseases, such as arthritis, have gotten worse and fail to recognize when depression is causing patients' deterioration.

To be fair, this can happen to anyone. Why? The symptoms of arthritis and depression are subjective. Doctors must rely upon patients' descriptions of how they feel to diagnose either. Unlike diabetes or chronic kidney disease, there are few objective indicators of either arthritis or depression to examine or test. Sure, there are x-rays and blood tests for arthritis, but it is how patients feel that counts. You'd be surprised how difficult it is for many people to describe exactly how they feel. Older adults, especially, often feel uncomfortable talking about emotional problems and couch complaints in physical terms, further clouding the picture.

Even when depression is evident, people's tendency to see depression in older adults as an expectable reaction to disease contributes to depression being dismissed. Daniel's family did not see his orneriness and loss of interest as warning signs of a serious health problem because they viewed them as understandable.

When I met Daniel it was clear to me that his biggest problem was depression. As I saw it, retirement had taken a bit of the wind out of his sails. It had whittled away at his can-do, self-assured spirit. This left him vulnerable when arthritis hit. He got pummeled emotionally, a little bit, day by day, until this triggered depression. The longer the depression went on, and the worse it got, the worse the arthritis became. A vicious cycle started and he spiraled downhill.

THE ARTHRITIS-DEPRESSION VICIOUS CYCLE

Depression and arthritis are both inflammatory conditions. Much like diabetes, the relationship between depression and arthritis is a two-way street. The inflammation arthritis causes can alter the activity of brain circuits, resulting in depression. Once depression takes hold, it causes its own inflammatory effects that stoke the flames of arthritis. You can see how a physiological vicious cycle gets established.

Behavioral factors then fan the flames, winding up this vicious cycle further. Successfully living with arthritis requires participation in physical therapy and regular exercise. It takes a lot of motivation to exercise when you are stiff and in pain. Depression robs patients of the ambition, energy, motivation, and determination necessary to make exercise part of their lifestyle.

Depression causes excess disability, another important concept in geriatrics. Excess disability refers to a level of added disability above and beyond that caused by a single disease. Depression accounts for much excess disability, and Daniel had more than his share. In his case, arthritis alone would have caused only minor restrictions of activity. In fact, he did not become severely disabled until depression overtook him.

Excess disability is common in arthritis sufferers who also have depression. Among patients with arthritis, the severity of their depression and pain predicts how much disability they have much better than the actual amount of joint damage visible on their x-rays. In other words, limitation of movement and function has less to do with the amount of actual joint damage and more to do with depressive emotions.[4]

INTERRUPTING THE VICIOUS CYCLE

In cases such as Daniel's, the key to improving well-being and function is interrupting the vicious cycle by treating depression. I diagnosed major depressive disorder and prescribed a selective serotonin reuptake inhibitor (SSRI) antidepressant for Daniel. Duloxetine (Cymbalta), a serotonin norepinephrine reuptake inhibitor (SNRI) antidepressant, is often touted as being especially good for depression and pain. It happens to be a very good medication, although not for everyone. In my experience, there is nothing magical about duloxetine for arthritis patients. Any antidepressant that relieves depression will also improve its associated pain and disability.

This proved true for Daniel. He had a good response to the SSRI antidepressant. His attitude and outlook improved, and he became interested in watching his grandchildren play soccer and baseball after school. He astonished his wife, pleasantly so, when, without fanfare, he got his golf clubs out of the cellar, carried them up the cellar stairs on his own, and drove himself to the driving range to hit balls. He found the results disappointing, but he sought out the course golf pro who showed him how to adjust his swing to lessen the arthritis pain. He could not hit drives more than 180 yards, but he began playing again and didn't let his diminished prowess bother him . . . too much.

Daniel had a very good result from antidepressant medication, but psychotherapy also works. One type of psychotherapy, cognitive behavioral therapy, can be helpful in reducing the negative thinking from depression that keeps older adults from adjusting to challenging aspects of aging, such as arthritis. Psychotherapy is not a purely mental treatment. Cognitive behavioral therapy reduces levels of interleukin-6 (IL-6), an inflammatory chemical that is elevated in arthritis and depression.[5]

Any psychotherapy that focuses on how patients cope with problems may help arthritis patients. Arthritis patients who tend to use denial to cope with problems or believe that nothing they can do will make a difference have more depression and pain. Such attitudes are very detrimental to coping with any health problem. Psychotherapy can help patients learn to see such thinking in themselves and adopt more positive ways of coping.

Arthritis sufferers have flare-ups from time to time. During these flare-ups, which are temporary, symptoms get worse. Depressed patients have a hard time recognizing flare-ups as passing states they can ride out. To the contrary, they react to flare-ups as if they are end-of-the-world tragedies. Such thinking becomes a self-fulfilling prophecy: pessimism, negativity, and doom-and-gloom thinking make the depression worse, and this fuels the vicious cycle, making the flare-up that much worse.

LAUGHTER IS THE BEST MEDICINE?

Arthritis is a good example of the power of the mind-brain-body connection. In addition to psychotherapy, mindfulness practices can have beneficial physical affects on arthritis. Mindfulness meditation may be effective in relieving pain and depression in patients with a depressive disorder who also have arthritis. The effect is not purely psychological. One study found that meditation reduced joint swelling and tenderness.[6]

We like to say that laughter is the best medicine, and there is some truth to it. One study showed that mirthful laughter reduced levels of inflammatory chemicals, such as IL-6, in some patients with rheumatoid arthritis.[7] I wonder how the scientists in that study distinguished mirthful laughing from run-of-the-mill chuckles. Wouldn't you also like to know what they did to make their subjects laugh mirthfully, especially those who were depressed? If I find out, I'll let you know in a second edition of this book.

Speaking of mirthful laughter, let's take a minute to check on how you, my readers, are doing. I often recommend books on Alzheimer's disease to the family caregivers of my patients. More often than not, they tell me that reading these books makes them feel depressed. You have read a good deal of this book, and I hope doing so has not made you depressed. My intention has been to warn you about depression. Warnings are never pleasant. But I have coupled the warning with a message of hope that you can take action to feel better, stay healthier, and live longer. And I want you to have facts that you need to take action. And while you're at it, make sure to have a good laugh.

13

DEPRESSION AND PARKINSON'S DISEASE

Until now we have focused on the effect depression has on organs of the body other than the brain. True, stroke is a brain disease, but it is actually a vascular disease that impacts the circulation in the brain, not the brain itself. In this chapter and the next we deal with diseases of the brain substance. Parkinson's and Alzheimer's are degenerative brain diseases. Degenerative brain diseases occur when brain cells die off. As more and more cells die, the brain deteriorates and the disease progresses. You may be familiar with the differences between Parkinson's and Alzheimer's. However, there are also important similarities between them, one being the impact of depression.

LORRAINE

Lorraine was a bookkeeper for a party goods company. She was married and had three children, and considered herself to be a pretty boring person. So did almost everyone she knew. Her personality was dour, pessimistic, negative, and always worried. She had no fun or joy in life. The glass in Lorraine's world was always half empty. She lived in dread, always expecting the worst.

If Lorraine reminds you of Juliette, the patient I described in chapter 7, it's because they both had dysthymia. Dysthymia is a chronic, low-grade form of depression. Because it is not usually debilitating, people live with dysthymia for long periods of time, sometimes most of their lives, without treatment. Such prolonged exposure makes dysthymia more destructive than major depression, which is more severe but (usually) much shorter lasting.

Fortunately for Lorraine, her health held up fairly well. It was not until age sixty-four that the first symptoms of Parkinson's came out. It started with shaking in her right arm. This gradually got worse and then spread to her left arm. Her face became less and less expressive and took on a staring look. This can make persons with Parkinson's disease seem unemotional, aloof, withdrawn, or depressed. But no one took much note of this change in Lorraine's appearance. Because of her dysthymia, people who knew her were used to her showing no emotion. Family members and friends did not make much of the general slowness of movement that soon came over her. She had never been an animated or lively person, so they interpreted this as just more of the same plus the effects of aging. But the tremor was a giveaway. At a yearly checkup, Lorraine's primary care physician spotted the tremor and other symptoms, and made a referral to a neurologist. The neurologist examined Lorraine and diagnosed Parkinson's disease. Hearing this, Lorraine concluded that the disaster she'd always expected had finally arrived. Feeling more hopeless and useless than ever, she decided to retire early.

STUCK IN MOLASSES

Imagine what it would feel like to be frozen—no, not like a popsicle, more like the tin man in *The Wizard of Oz*, locked inside a body in slow motion. Everything slows down: movement, speaking, and even thinking. Your ideas seem shut out in the cold, searching for an open door into your mind. Once you know what you want to say, your mouth hesitates to speak the words. You try to walk, but your feet seem magnetized to the floor. Once you manage to get started, it may be hard to stop or change direction. You fall down without warning. Your speech is soft and mumbling. Others struggle to understand you.

In addition to your body not moving when you want it to, there are extra movements you do not want. When you are still, you tremble. People see this and think you must be nervous. You feel restless much of the time. And the medications your neurologist gave you to help your

Parkinson's disease make you twitch and writhe some of the time. Struggling with a body that does not obey your commands is stressful, and you often feel anxious or depressed.

This is how it feels to have Parkinson's. I've never experienced it, so I do not speak from personal experience. But I've treated many patients with the disease and listened to their anguished descriptions of how it feels. Frustration, anger, insecurity, embarrassment, and self-pity are common reactions to life with this disease.

Those Parkinson's patients who seek my help do so because of more severe mental health problems. Some have dementia. Others have hallucinations (seeing or hearing things that are not there) or delusions (false, irrational beliefs) caused by their anti-Parkinson's medications. But depression is, by far, the most common psychiatric complication.

In chapter 3 we looked at how Parkinson's can cause depression. In this chapter we'll see that depression might cause Parkinson's and definitely makes it worse.

CAN DEPRESSION CAUSE PARKINSON'S DISEASE?

Studies tell us that patients who develop Parkinson's often have had depression previously. This pattern could signify two possibilities. First, depression might be a risk factor for Parkinson's. Risks factors are conditions that increase the chance of getting a disease. Smoking is a risk factor for emphysema. In other words, having depression may increase your chance of getting Parkinson's. But, second, it also could mean that depression is a prodrome of Parkinson's disease.[1] Prodromes are preliminary manifestations of a condition. Sometimes they appear right before the onset of a condition, but in other cases there can be a gap of months or years. This means that depression could be the earliest sign of Parkinson's, just as chronic cough might be a prodrome of emphysema in a smoker.

One study looked at patients who had depression five to nine years before they got Parkinson's. The researchers assumed that five to nine years was too long a separation between depression and Parkinson's for depression to be a prodrome, so it had to be a risk factor. The results tell an interesting story. People who had depression had triple the rate of Parkinson's disease, five to nine years later, than those without depression. The conclusion was that previous depression is a risk factor for developing Parkinson's disease.[2] The results of this study also show that the older you are when you get depression, and the more severe or hard to treat your depression turns out to be, the more likely you are to get Parkinson's.

So was Lorraine's history of dysthymic depression a factor in her getting Parkinson's disease? Maybe, but there is no way to know in an individual person. Research tells us what happens on average. Perhaps the more thought-provoking question is, "Had she been treated for depression years earlier, and gotten better, might she have avoided Parkinson's disease?" Again, there is no way to know yet. More research is needed.

But here's the thing: right now there is good evidence to suspect that depression earlier in life puts people at risk for Parkinson's later in life. Knowing this, are you still reluctant to have treatment for depression? Do you really want to gamble with the health of your brain?

WHAT IS PARKINSON'S DISEASE?

Before we go on, let's take a moment to understand Parkinson's in more detail. Parkinson's is a movement disorder. It is classified this way, because its distinguishing symptoms involve bodily movement. The main symptoms of Parkinson's are tremor (shaking), stiffness (rigidity), and slowness of movement (called bradykinesia). Those affected often have stooped posture, shuffling gait, soft or mumbling speech, poor balance, and a blank expression. Falls are common and lead to injuries. Parkinson's is a chronic and progressive movement disorder. It gradually worsens over time, and no treatment prevents this, although treatment eases the symptoms.

I've noticed that patients and family members find movement disorders confusing. Some movement disorders, including Huntington's disease and tardive dyskinesia, cause involuntary movements that are more irregular, twitching and writhing in appearance. As I mentioned earlier, medications for Parkinson's cause these abnormal movements as side effects. They are different from Parkinson's abnormal movements, which are tremors consisting of highly rhythmic shaking.

Another source of confusion is that not all causes of Parkinsonism are due to Parkinson's disease. Poor circulation in the brain can cause atherosclerotic Parkinsonism. Other causes of Parkinsonism include certain medications, carbon monoxide poisoning, and repeated head trauma.

The difference between Parkinson's and other diseases that cause Parkinsonism is that Parkinson's is a degenerative brain disease. Degenerative brain diseases are illnesses in which brain cells become sick and die. When enough cells are lost, the brain circuits they serve begin to malfunction and symptoms appear. Parkinson's primarily involves brain circuits involved in movement. But as the degeneration progresses, the symptoms get worse and worse and other parts of the brain are affected, including those involved in emotions, thinking, and behavior. If you are reading this chapter out of particular interest in Parkinson's, you may have heard of Lewy body disease, a degenerative dementia similar to Alzheimer's that also causes Parkinsonism.

Parkinson's is the second most common degenerative brain disease after Alzheimer's. It affects 1 to 2 percent of those over sixty-five years of age, worldwide, which amounts to over one million individuals in the United States.[3]

PARKINSON'S DISEASE AND DEPRESSION: A CHICKEN-AND-EGG PROBLEM

As you can imagine, developing Parkinson's didn't do anything to make Lorraine less depressed—just the opposite. This crushing development fed right into her gloom-and-doom outlook on life. Then her chronic dysthymia morphed into a severe major depression. She had always been down in the dumps and downcast, but now she was hopeless and distraught and lost interest in doing anything. Many days she didn't bother to get dressed or get out of bed. Parkinson's disease can be disabling, but Lorraine had been taken over by depression.

That being the case, Parkinson's still occupied the center of medical attention initially. Lorraine's neurologist prescribed medications that helped for a while. They lessened the shaking, but eventually it came back and got worse. Lorraine's movements became slower, and her gait took on a shuffling quality. Once or twice she fell after catching her heels on the rug.

As the Parkinson's became more disabling, Lorraine's neurologist tried to stem the tide with more complicated medication regimens, but the results were disappointing. I wasn't surprised when I heard this. In my experience, severely depressed Parkinson's patients do not get much better neurologically until their depression is treated. The flip side of this observation is that once the depression does get better, the Parkinson's symptoms also improve, usually without any additional treatment.

Once Lorraine took to bed, her husband became much more worried. She was quickly becoming a complete invalid. In horror, he feared she would soon end up in a nursing home. Lorraine was now only sixty-eight years old, and that was when he brought her to see me.

Depression is very common among patients with Parkinson's. Forty to sixty percent may have it.[4] One reason we are not exactly sure of the number is that depression can be hard to recognize among patients who already have Parkinson's because the two conditions share so many symptoms. The overlap of affected brain circuits accounts for this. Apathy, lack of motivation, low energy levels, slowness of movement and thinking, soft speech, lack of outward emotional expression, loss of interest, difficulty concentrating, poor appetite, weight loss, and sleep disturbance are seen in both illnesses. In contrast, sadness, undue pessimism, absence of pleasure in living, irritability, anxiety, and suicidal thoughts point more to depression.[5]

When depression strikes a person with Parkinson's disease it speeds up the deterioration. Motor function, cognitive ability, and overall disability worsen. Patients with depression need anti-Parkinson's medications sooner than patients with Parkinson's who are not depressed.[6] And caregivers experience a dramatic increase in stress and strain.[7] Depression turns out to be more troubling and burdensome than the Parkinsonism.[8]

Lorraine's is a classic chicken-and-egg dilemma. Was her lifelong dysthymic depression a factor in her getting Parkinson's disease? Maybe so. Once she got Parkinson's, her depression became much worse. Was this a psychological reaction to being diagnosed with a terrible disease? Possibly. But just as likely, Parkinson's further damaged the mood circuits in her brain. Either way, the deepening depression caused the Parkinson's to advance faster and become more debilitating.

If your head is spinning, that seems about right because we are going around and around in another vicious cycle between depression and a disease. Depression and Parkinson's share overlapping brain circuits and brain chemistry. One makes the other worse and vice versa.

PSYCHIATRIC TREATMENT TO THE RESCUE

Fortunately, depression in patients with Parkinson's disease responds to treatment. It is thus truly tragic that fewer than half of those with depression receive treatment for it.[9] Antidepressants work. So does cognitive behavioral therapy, a form of psychotherapy, or what people call counseling.[10] Successful treatment of depression not only helps to improve emotional well-being and function but also improves the movement symptoms, function, and overall quality of life.

I treated Lorraine with an antidepressant medication and helped her family learn how to be more effective in helping her overcome her negative thinking and pessimism. Eventually she got better, although her improvement was far from miraculous. Treatment lessened her depression but only back to the level of her lifelong dysthymia. Nonetheless she got out of bed, started taking care of herself again, and became more functional. Her Parkinson's symptoms lessened too, and her neurologist was able to lower the doses of her medications.

NEUROINFLAMMATION: A COMMON LINK?

With the completion of this chapter, we've now seen the role depression plays in a number of diseases associated with aging. Maybe you've even felt that the chapters are beginning to sound like the same old story. Good, because there are common threads tying them together. Inflammation is one, and it is the basis of one theory of aging called inflamm-aging.[11]

According to this theory, the lifelong, cumulative, damaging effects of chronic inflammation are responsible for the telltale signs of aging and the common diseases that go with it. Depression, as we now well know, is more than just a disorder of mood; it also is a state of heightened inflammation, feeding into inflamm-aging, adding insult to injury, and thus speeding up the aging process.

Inflammation occurring in the nervous system, including the brain, is called neuroinflammation.[12] Depression increases the level of inflammation in the brain as well as in the rest of the body. In so doing, depression, a brain disease, accelerates brain aging, and this hastens the onset of degenerative brain diseases.

Parkinson's may be one example. Alzheimer's is probably another. It's not that depression causes these diseases per se. Depression, and the extended stress response it triggers, lets loose a barrage of inflammation and oxidative damage.[13] Combine these destructive forces with genetic and environmental factors and, voilà, your brain ages faster and you get brain diseases earlier.

Imagine owning a ten-year-old car that you've cared for well. Maybe you've parked it in a garage and tried not to drive it in bad weather. It might have sixty thousand miles on it, but it looks and runs like new, and it's not given you a bit of trouble. But now circumstances change and you have to park it outside, in harsh weather. And you must drive it rain or shine over poorly maintained roads full of potholes you can't avoid. Before long, your car no longer looks new, and things start to break. After ten thousand miles of such automotive stress, your car, which still has only 70,000 miles on it, now looks old and worn out, like a car with 120,000 miles. Depression puts hard miles on your body. It makes you old before your time and might mean the difference between getting Parkinson's disease in your sixties instead of in your seventies. That difference is a very big deal.

CONCLUSION

Depression is very common among persons with Parkinson's disease. In some cases depression comes on after Parkinson's, in other cases before. We know that depression makes Parkinson's worse. It increases the severity of the symptoms and causes it to progress faster. Treatment of depression lessens misery, neurological symptoms, and disability in Parkinson's, as it did in Lorraine's case. If you have Parkinson's and also suffer from depression, I hope I have convinced you to get treatment for the depression. It's a no-brainer to take care of your brain.

And if you do not have Parkinson's but do have depression, here's another reason not to ignore it. Treatment of depression might stave off a degenerative brain disease such as Parkinson's. If you have not known anyone with Parkinson's, take it from me, this is a chance to prevent an illness you definitely do not want to get.

14

DEPRESSION AND ALZHEIMER'S DISEASE

Think about this: what if depression increases your chance of getting Alzheimer's disease?

Have you found it incredible that depression might be a factor in so many serious illnesses? Maybe you are thinking "not Alzheimer's too!" Yes, I am afraid so. Untreated depression greatly increases the chance of getting Alzheimer's and other types of dementia. In this chapter I'm going to focus just on Alzheimer's. It's the most common cause of dementia, and we know the most about it.

With good reason, older adults dread the prospect of this disease. Most would do nearly anything to avoid it. My patients, and their middle-age children, constantly ask me whether any new treatments are available. They hope against hope that I will answer yes, and they would jump at the chance to take a new treatment.

Yet many have a very different attitude about depression. They shun treatment for depression like the plague, preferring to live with it instead. They shouldn't! Not without understanding that ignoring depression increases their chances of getting Alzheimer's. DEPRESSION DOUBLES YOUR RISK FOR ALZHEIMER'S DISEASE. That's right, you read that correctly. Depression doubles the risk of Alzheimer's!

When it comes to mental health and aging, Alzheimer's gets all the public attention. But depression is just as big a problem, maybe bigger. One in nine older adults has Alzheimer's, but one in five has clinically significant depression.[1] Both brain diseases cause misery, disability, and anguish for families. The negative attitude toward depression is a shame because depression can be treated and Alzheimer's cannot. But the tragic irony, as I've already pointed out, is that depression leads to Alzheimer's.

When I recommend treatment to my patients with depression, all too often my advice seems to fall on deaf ears. Or they look as if I'm offering them a root canal without novocaine. A polite "thanks, but no thanks" is what I hear, in one form or another. But when I then tell the same patients that depression can cause Alzheimer's, I have their attention.

LESTER

Lester was an eighty-three-year-old widower. He had been a middle manager in a midsize office supplies company. He enjoyed practical jokes, kidding around, and making puns. When I met Lester, he'd been struggling with depression for ten months.

Lester had moderately severe depression. He felt down, felt no pleasure in anything, didn't care about what happened to him, and wasn't doing a good job taking care of himself. But he wasn't debilitated. He was barely treading water but had not gone under, yet.

Despite his depression, Lester was still able to kid around with me. Before even shaking my hand in the reception area of my office, he demanded to know, in front of several other patients, whether I believed I was worth everything Medicare was paying me. If you have any familiarity with what Medicare pays geriatric psychiatrists these days, you realize this was no joke to me. I laughed anyway and told him I hoped so. I also suggested that if he felt unsatisfied with his visit he could write his congressman to suggest the government try to get its money back. Lester loved my willingness to play along with him, and this helped him warm up to me and got our relationship off to a good start.

As often happens in my practice, it was Lester's son, Rick, who had made Lester's appointment for him. Lester really didn't want any part of it but humored his son. Rick was quite concerned about Lester's depression. As Rick put it, his dad seemed to be "going downhill fast." Lester described his mood as "in the toilet." He was gloomy, negative and pessimistic, felt he'd gotten too old, and saw no point in getting any older. He wasn't suicidal but admitted he'd be happy to die in his sleep.

I thought Lester had major depressive disorder and recommended treatment. Literally, "thanks, Doc, but no thanks" was his reply. This was followed by "no offense, Doc, but I don't believe in it." Lester took a liking to me and was trying to cushion the blow. Lester did not believe in psychiatric treatment. He firmly believed that people ought to be able to handle their feelings on their own. He said he appreciated how hard I was trying to help him and, teasing me further, promised to write his congressman with instructions to have Medicare pay me more.

Let me pause here for a moment to talk about an important point that Lester illustrates. Older patients with depression do not always look the way we expect patients with depression to look. We touched on this in chapter 4. Lester was kidding around. Had he not fessed up to his symptoms, there was little in my encounter with him to tip me off to his depression—quite the opposite. He was outwardly gregarious and seemed upbeat. Depression in older adults often looks different than we expect, and healthcare professionals must rely on observations of those close to the patient to get the whole picture, as I did with Rick.

As we will see in chapter 17, it often takes some effort to convince older adults to accept treatment for depression. Having told me to get lost, in a good-natured way, Lester seemed proud of himself. It was as if he'd gotten rid of a pesky door-to-door salesman. (No offense to older readers who may have earned their living as door-to-door salesmen.) Remember those days?

Like a successful salesman, I didn't give up easily on making a sale. I got my foot in the proverbial door. I told Lester I was sorry and disappointed that there was nothing I could do for him. Then I asked whether he would be interested in a treatment that could keep him from getting Alzheimer's. He looked at me skeptically but told me, as a matter of fact, he would.

Lester had seen what Alzheimer's did to his mother and brother. He watched helplessly as it robbed them of who they were, turning them into shells of their former selves. He wanted no part of this and had thought he'd kill himself to avoid a similar fate. In fact, I detected mild short-term and word retrieval problems, and I worried that depression was already dragging Lester down the path to Alzheimer's.

I explained to Lester the connection between depression and Alzheimer's disease. He listened seriously, without joking or kidding around, and he agreed to let me treat him for depression. I prescribed 50 mg of sertraline daily, and it worked well. Lester's depression got better, and his memory and language abilities improved.

I continued to see Lester every few months, and four years later Lester was still well, with no depression and no sign of Alzheimer's—a real success story.

DON'T STICK YOUR HEAD IN THE SAND

By the time most adults reach middle age, Alzheimer's disease is on their radar screens. If you are thirty, and you forget where you parked your car, you don't give it a second thought. But the first time it happens after you have turned sixty, your first thought will be, "Uh oh, it's starting."

Almost everyone knows or has known someone with Alzheimer's, and most everyone knows at least something about the disease.[2] But very few people know enough. And no one knows that depression can increase the risk of getting Alzheimer's. Since I began working on this book, I have not encountered a single person—not one—who knew that depression doubles the chance of Alzheimer's. I want to make sure that my readers know it.

Depression exerts its role in causing Alzheimer's disease throughout life.[3] I mentioned earlier that having depression doubles the risk for Alzheimer's. But depression very early in life is much worse. It quadruples the risk of Alzheimer's. The more episodes of depression you have over your lifetime, and the more severe they are, the greater the risk.[4]

Maybe you are reading this book because you are concerned about an elderly parent with depression. Maybe depression runs in your family. Maybe you also have a thirtysomething son or daughter with untreated depression. Guess what? You have good reason to worry about your parent and your child. They should both have treatment for depression.

We can't prevent Alzheimer's. But we can stave it off. Exercising, eating a Mediterranean diet, and keeping your weight down are all things you can do to lessen your risk. Treating depression is another. If you are sixty-five years old, you have a 10 percent chance of developing

Alzheimer's during the rest of your life. If you have untreated depression, you just doubled your risk!

I have spent over thirty years talking to patients and family members about Alzheimer's disease. I have noticed that, in general, people know Alzheimer's is bad, but they are often not aware of how bad it can be. If you have depression, and still do not plan on having treatment for it, you better know what you might be letting yourself in for. Let's have a serious look.

ALZHEIMER'S DISEASE: NOT A PRETTY PICTURE

Most people think of Alzheimer's as a memory disorder that causes forgetfulness for events, information, names, faces, how to do things, and where to find things. They recognize that it can rob victims of their independence. Even scarier is the threat of forgetting pieces of your own identity or the possibility of not knowing your loved ones any longer. This possibility horrifies the vast majority of people.

No doubt memory is important. But Alzheimer's is much more than just a memory disorder. It affects every facet of life. In my experience, if you haven't lived with or cared for someone with severe Alzheimer's you probably do not realize how awful it can be. Let me describe it for you.

Alzheimer's progresses through stages, mild, moderate, severe, and profound. It begins with barely noticeable forgetfulness. People often misplace common objects or forget names of persons they have known for a long time. Most people tell themselves this is just normal aging and try not to worry. But it gradually worsens. Problems become apparent to others, and all kinds of blunders start to happen. Getting lost, losing money, or forgetting to pay bills are just a few of the possible mishaps that plague those in the mild stage. A gnawing insecurity may set in, and patients often withdraw from familiar activities, which start to feel inexplicably baffling. Anxiety and depression are common at this stage.

As the disease enters the moderate stage, patients become unable to recall events as they occur. They start to forget details of their own lives, such as their address or telephone number or the town they are from. They still know the names of close family members, whom they depend on more and more to feel safe and secure. Patients may be afraid to be alone and insist family members stay with them all the time. These patients shadow family members around the house constantly. They may become frantic if their caregiver goes into the bathroom alone. This very quickly becomes unbearably stressful for caregivers.

Patients with moderate Alzheimer's usually cannot travel independently. A few individuals still drive and miraculously somehow find their way to very familiar, local destinations (e.g., neighborhood supermarket). I always cringe when I find out that a patient with moderate Alzheimer's still drives. It reminds me of the old driving safety slogan "watch out for the other guy." Family members lose sleep worrying about these patients' driving, but many can't bring themselves to take the car keys away.

At this stage patients cannot survive long without help. Left to their own devices, they may eat poorly and irregularly. Accidents, such as kitchen fires, easily occur. My patients have put metal objects in the microwave oven, tried to dry laundry in the oven (set on broil), and eaten rotten food. Usually they need help to pick out clothing and dress properly. They do not remember to shower or bathe and often do not change their clothing for days.

Patients in the moderate stage need much day-to-day help but do not recognize that something is wrong. Their caregivers' attempts to help feel intrusive and unnatural. Patients sometimes react belligerently. Others become more withdrawn and may have serious depression.

Entry into the severe stage is a turning point for family members because the severe stage demands more of them, physically and emotionally. Affected individuals seem less and less like themselves. They have trouble recalling details of their own life stories. They start to forget who relatives are, or develop delusions that relatives are impostors or doubles, or that they mean them harm. They become unaware of their surroundings and situation, and will need help with dressing, showering, and using the toilet. Incontinence occurs and can be a big problem. Patients may urinate or defecate anywhere, furniture, closets, drawers, and so forth. If they make it to the bathroom, they may make a big mess. Agitated or violent behavior becomes more common. Sleep disturbances are frequent. Patients often sleep during the day and are up at night. This disrupts the household.

As depressing as this sounds, it gets worse. In the profound, or advanced, stage, all or almost all abilities are lost. The person may no longer speak or walk. Days are spent in bed or sitting in a chair doing nothing and not uttering a word. They may have to be fed and may have trouble swallowing solid foods. In this state, patients no longer have much awareness, if any, of themselves or their surroundings.

Alzheimer's disease has been described as death by inches. You can probably appreciate why. Afflicted individuals slip away, bit by bit, each day. In the earlier stages the person with Alzheimer's suffers more. Later on, it's their family members who suffer.

Taking care of a loved one with Alzheimer's takes a toll on family caregivers. Caregivers experience chronic stress and exhaustion. Many become depressed. And most alarming, the chronic stress and depression of caregiving increases the chance that the caregiver will get Alzheimer's. Knowing that depression increases the chance of all this, will you still think twice about having treatment? Really?

HOW DOES DEPRESSION DO IT?

Much like Parkinson's, the relationship between depression and Alzheimer's is complicated. Early on, depression can occur as an emotional reaction to facing the rest of one's life with Alzheimer's. Later in the course of the disease, depression may be caused by damage Alzheimer's does to mood-regulating circuits in the brain. Sometimes these circuits are affected earliest, and depression occurs before the more familiar symptoms of Alzheimer's appear. In other words, depression can be the earliest symptom of Alzheimer's. Now—this may be confusing—if you get depression years or decades before Alzheimer's has begun, depression might not be the earliest symptom of the disease; it might be the cause!

Scientists are beginning to piece together the puzzle of how depression might cause Alzheimer's. The most widely accepted theory today is that Alzheimer's patients make excessive amounts of a protein called amyloid beta. This protein accumulates in the brain, where it forms the plaques that are one of the hallmarks of Alzheimer's. High levels of amyloid beta are toxic to brain cells. Inflammation and oxidative damage may explain this in part. As you know, depression also heightens inflammation and oxidative damage, compounding the toxicity of amyloid beta.

Depression also increases levels of amyloid beta in the brain. This occurs even with depression among younger adults. So decades of excessive amyloid beta causes Alzheimer's, and depression exposes the brain to higher levels earlier in life. Each episode of prolonged depression amounts to another exposure to toxic amyloid beta. In essence, depression gives Alzheimer's a head start (no pun intended).[5]

Depression also causes a reduction of brain-derived neurotrophic factor, or BDNF, which, you will recall, is a brain maintenance protein. Without enough BDNF, new brain cells do not sprout in the hippocampus and it starts to shrink. This mimics what happens in early Alzheimer's. Short-term memory begins to fail. Depression also elevates levels of the stress hormone cortisol, which also causes the hippocampus to shrink. In other areas of the brain, the lack of BDNF means that many fewer new nerve cell connections form. The brain begins to wither, and cognitive ability slips. The longer the depression goes on, the worse this gets.

Depression amounts to a brain drain. It drains brain reserve capacity.[6] Think of brain reserve capacity as being akin to your retirement funds. The larger your nest egg and the slower you spend it, the longer you can maintain your lifestyle in retirement. The less you start out with and the faster you spend it, the sooner you'll be in the poorhouse. Prior depression makes you spend some of your retirement money before you retire, so you have a smaller nest egg, and Alzheimer's also makes you spend it faster once you retire so you wind up in the neurologic poorhouse.

DEPRESSION AND PASCAL'S WAGER? HEADS YOU WIN, TAILS YOU GET ALZHEIMER'S DISEASE

Can we say definitely that depression causes Alzheimer's? No, we can't say this beyond a shadow of a doubt, but the evidence is hard to ignore. What about treatment for depression? Does it prevent Alzheimer's? Again, we do not know. Are you willing to gamble that it does not?

The seventeenth-century philosopher Blaise Pascal said that everybody gambles with their lives in their decisions regarding whether or not to believe in God. His famous "wager" goes like this: If God exists, and you choose not to believe, then you risk damnation. On the other hand, if God does not exist, and you do believe, then you have little to lose except for the time and energy you spent worshipping. The safe "bet" is to believe.

In the same vein, if depression does cause Alzheimer's and you do not have treatment, you double (or worse) your chance of getting the disease. Conversely, if depression does not cause Alzheimer's but you get treatment, you don't lose, because you will get your life back. You'll feel like yourself again, be healthier, and live longer. Having treatment for depression is the smarter "wager."

CONCLUSION

We face a worldwide epidemic of Alzheimer's disease. Alzheimer's is a personal tragedy for the millions of individuals affected and tens of millions of their family members and friends. It also is a global economic catastrophe. In the United Sates alone Alzheimer's already costs three hundred billion dollars per year. By 2050 it will cost over a trillion dollars—just in the United States! This is an emergency for which the world is not prepared.[7] As of yet we have no cure, or even good treatments to slow it down. Anything that can be done to stave it off will help a lot. Treating depression is one such thing.[8]

15

DEPRESSION CAN BE A REAL PAIN: DEPRESSION AND PAIN

Do you have chronic pain? If you are an older adult, chances are you do. If you are younger, chronic pain may be waiting for you in the future. Startled by these statements? Here's a fact you may find surprising: more than half of older people living at home endure chronic pain.[1]

Chronic pain is defined as pain that lasts more than six months. Excluding pain related to cancer, the major types of chronic pain are musculoskeletal and neuropathic.[2] Musculoskeletal pain originates in bones and muscles, back and joint problems making up the vast majority. Frequent causes include osteoarthritis, osteoporosis, spinal stenosis, fibromyalgia, and degenerative disk disease. Neuropathic pain comes from diseases that damage nerves or affect their function. Diabetes, shingles, alcoholism, and injury are some of the causes of neuropathic pain.

Many individuals manage chronic pain well, experiencing little impact from it. For many others, chronic pain worsens their quality of life. As you can imagine, chronic pain can unravel lives and cause indescribable agony. Chronic pain forces sufferers to give up household, occupational, and recreational activities, and it can be extremely disabling. Victims' lives become more narrow and restricted, and they may become socially isolated. Those disabled by their pain lose independence and self-esteem.

Living with prolonged pain can be emotionally trying. About half of persons with chronic pain suffer from depression.[3] The relationship between chronic pain and depression is complicated. Chronic pain can be depressing. But the relationship goes both ways. Depression can bring on chronic pain, make the pain more severe, or prevent treatment from relieving it.

CHRONIC PAIN IS COMPLEX PAIN

Everyone, even toddlers, understands acute pain. Human accident proneness ensures this. Stub your toe, bang your head, or close a drawer on your finger, and you get it, literally and figuratively.

Acute pain is simple. Injury or some type of physical disturbance, somewhere in your body, generates pain signals, from the origin, that we feel as pain. Usually the cause is identifiable. Medical treatment, when needed, involves physical approaches to ease the pain and relieve the problem.

Chronic pain is much more complex. Proper evaluation and treatment requires a multipronged approach that goes beyond the physical to include the emotional, cognitive, functional, and social dimensions of chronic pain.[4] Healthcare services are not generally set up for this. My experience has been that older adults' chronic pain is most often approached from a fairly narrow physical perspective. The treatments they receive are usually limited to pain medications, physical therapy, steroid injections, nerve blocks, and surgery. These approaches can work well, but many patients need more.

Those who are also depressed need more. Even though half of chronic-pain patients suffer from depression, their depression is rarely addressed.[5] Family members often dismiss depression as an expectable reaction to pain. "Why wouldn't they be depressed, living with all that pain?" is an explanation I hear frequently for why they feel their relative does not need treatment for depression. This sentiment reflects two incorrect beliefs about old age. The first is that pain is an inevitable part of aging. One of my patients once told me, "It [pain] comes with the deal." The second is that depression is a normal reaction to being old and all that goes with it. Neither idea about old age is correct, but both lead people to suffer needlessly rather than get help. We looked at such beliefs, in detail, in chapter 1.

Depression is not a normal or expectable reaction to chronic pain. Many older adults with chronic pain do not get depression. But when depression is present, it is not to be taken lightly. Depression adds to the hopelessness and uselessness that chronic-pain patients feel and makes them even more socially withdrawn and isolated. And one in five patients with chronic pain feel suicidal.[6]

Unfortunately, patients too often do not disclose that they are depressed. Even when others see their depression, patients may not accept help for it. We have seen this pattern in previous chapters, affecting older adults with a range of healthcare problems.

Chronic-pain patients worry that once they are labeled with a psychiatric problem their pain will no longer be taken seriously.[7] Such fears are too often well founded. When physicians cannot find a physical cause to explain pain or account for its severity, or pain does not respond as expected to one of the therapies I mentioned before, they are wont to blame emotional factors. This is easy to do when depression is present because it is widely known that depression causes aches and pains.

Once doctors determine that depression is a factor in chronic pain, many lose interest. Patients sense this. I see the reactions of those chronic-pain patients referred to me. Even when I personally know that the referring doctors have continued to be highly interested and actively involved in their patients' care, their patients nevertheless arrive at my office feeling emotionally banished. Many think that their doctors no longer believe their pain to be "real." They feel rejected and abandoned, and I must work hard to help them understand that just because there may be emotional and behavioral aspects to their pain, it does not mean their pain is not real or that there is not a physical cause for it.

GEORGETTE'S PAIN IN THE NECK

Georgette was a seventy-eight-year-old retired medical receptionist. She had been married to Burt for fifty-six years. Georgette had been fairly healthy until a few years earlier, when she developed neck pain. She took ibuprofen, an over-the-counter nonsteroidal anti-inflammatory agent (NSAID). But the pain didn't go away, and instead spread to her shoulders and head.

The primary care physician got an x-ray of Georgette's neck, which showed osteoarthritis. She prescribed a prescription-strength NSAID. This also didn't help, and neither did tramadol, a slightly stronger analgesic. The next step was a mild narcotic painkiller, but this also proved ineffective. Because of the pain, Georgette couldn't sleep, and she quit her volunteer work in the town library. Georgette began to feel discouraged and asked her doctor for something stronger. But her doctor was duly cautious. Rather than prescribe a stronger narcotic, she referred Georgette to an orthopedic surgeon.

The orthopedist's examination seemed very thorough, and Georgette felt hopeful that relief was at hand. He sent Georgette for an MRI scan of the neck. After reading the scan, the orthopedist referred Georgette for physical therapy. This seemed reasonable to Burt, but Georgette was skeptical. She didn't see what good this would do and now felt disappointed and frustrated as well as discouraged.

Physical therapy did not go well. Georgette found it painful and thought it made her worse. She participated halfheartedly or canceled appointments. Georgette became increasingly down and negative, and fell into utter despair. Frequent crying spells and hopelessness set in. She couldn't eat. At times of greatest distress, she cried out in anguish and agony, startling Burt. Was pain filling her with anguish, or was anguish making the pain worse?

As Georgette's pain worsened, Burt was more and more attentive to her. He took over the cooking and spared no effort in trying to make things she would eat. He was always at the ready with hot packs, cold packs, special pillows, neck massages, foot massages, and pain pills, and rarely strayed from her side lest she need something.

Seeing little progress, the physical therapist recommended a pain clinic to Georgette. The pain specialist was an anesthesiologist. Most people associate anesthesiologists with surgery, but some subspecialize in pain management. The anesthesiologist tried steroid injections. Sometimes these provided relief for a few days; other times they seemed to make things worse. Burt saw no rhyme or reason to it. Next came nerve blocks followed by Botox. Nothing helped.

In a very matter-of-fact way, the anesthesiologist told Georgette that there was no point in her coming back because he had nothing more to offer her. Something about his tone of voice made her feel guilty for not allowing him to succeed. Burt found the whole predicament very disturbing. He had been a mechanical engineer and was used to working with systems that made sense and operated logically. He had been paid to fix problems and couldn't understand why all these highly trained specialists could not fix Georgette's. He began searching the Internet looking for remedies and sought second and third opinions from a wide range of specialists. One consultant, on hearing Georgette's tale of woe, suggested that Georgette needed to see a psychiatrist. Burt was skeptical, but they had exhausted other options. He convinced Georgette to give it a try and found my name in the phone book.

The best pain clinics use a team approach that includes mental health specialists, often a psychiatrist and a social worker. My experience has been that most pain clinics have anesthesiologists, neurologists, orthopedists, and possibly rehabilitation specialists but rarely include mental health professionals, and social and mental health factors are not given adequate consideration. Pain is dealt with entirely as a physical problem, and any apparent emotional distress is assumed to be a normal reaction to the pain.

Georgette reluctantly agreed to see me, but she felt "they" had given up on her. When I met Georgette she looked absolutely pathetic. Her face was fixed in a grimace, and her brow was knit. Every few minutes she winced in pain and murmured "ouch." She had sudden spasms, as if an electric shock went through her. When this happened the "ouch" was yelled. I jumped the first time she did this. Before I said much of anything, Georgette began crying, and whimpered, "They think it's all in my head, but it's real!" I thought, "It's real, all right. The pain-depression complex has really got her good."

As I listened to Georgette and Burt each in turn describe the problem, a few things became obvious. First, Georgette had severe major depressive disorder, and this needed to be treated or little else would help. Second, the hour-by-hour challenge to deal with pain was all consuming for the couple. Chronic pain had become a way of life. And, third, what appeared on the surface to be a happy marriage was far from perfect.

Georgette and Burt had a stable, harmonious relationship and had treated each other respectfully. But Georgette had lived with some misgivings from the outset. Burt was a good provider and always made it home for dinner with the family. But he had outside interests—no, not that kind! He had been active in town politics and most evenings was at one committee meeting or another, or running for this or that office. He was never home. He had been a good father and had always been there for their children. But even when he was around, he seemed emotionally removed from Georgette. She had always felt low man on the totem pole of Burt's attention. Early on she'd made her peace with it, but for some reason in recent years it had begun to gnaw at her.

Now Burt hovered. He was always there dealing with the pain. But he still wasn't that emotionally supportive. Sometimes he even criticized her for being so dramatic or being a baby about it. He thought she ought to be more stoic. But Georgette had his full attention around the clock.

THE PAIN-DEPRESSION COMPLEX

Why does one person develop severe arthritis and learn to live with it while another, whose arthritis is no worse, becomes crippled with chronic pain from it? Depression often makes the difference. It did for Georgette. Depression caused a minor neck problem to snowball into a life-changing catastrophe. The interweaving of chronic pain and depression is called the pain-depression complex or the pain-depression syndrome.

In some cases, pain begins, more or less, as a purely physical problem. As it goes on unabated, and becomes chronic, it can easily trigger depression. But you do not have to have the pain first. Sometimes it's the other way around. Depression comes first and paves the way for pain. Older adults with depression have been shown to be more likely to develop pain than older persons without depression.[8]

In Georgette's case, it's not completely clear which came first, depression or chronic pain. At first glance it seemed that chronic pain came first and brought on the depression. But something earlier had first caused her to feel disturbed by aspects of her relationship with Burt that had not bothered her in many, many years. Could it have been a low-grade depression?

It is important to recognize that this can happen. But in Georgette's case it really doesn't matter. All that is really important is that she has both chronic pain and depression and both are severe. Once the pain-depression complex is established, pain makes depression worse and depression makes pain worse, and it goes around and around in a vicious cycle.

PAIN IS IN YOUR BRAIN

When you touch a hot pot, a reflex makes you pull your hand away even before you realize what happened. Not until the signals reach your brain do you become conscious of discomfort. Have you ever wondered why pain hurts? Our brains make pain a very unhappy experience for us so we'll learn to avoid it whenever we can. Pain causes emotional distress. It makes children cry, and many grown-ups, too. If you think about it, you may agree that pain shares a number of features with depression. Some specialists even believe that chronic pain may be a form of depression.[9]

The brain circuits responsible for creating the experience of pain overlap with the mood circuits affected in depression. Similar areas of the brain are involved, and the monoamine neurotransmitters, dopamine, serotonin, and norepinephrine, are affected in both. High levels of inflammation and oxidative stress are present in both as well.[10]

People with depression often experience various aches and pains that have no physical cause and that go away once the depression is treated. Why does this happen? The brain has the ability to adjust our perception of pain. This capacity helps us not feel pain if we are injured during an emergency. Depression does the opposite. It heightens sensitivity to pain. This can make ordinary signals from the body feel painful, or greatly amplify actual pain so it feels much more severe.

Attitude also makes a difference. People who remain confident that they can control their lives are far less prone to chronic pain. In contrast, pessimism, negativity, and lack of self-confidence, all symptoms of depression, characterize the thinking of those with chronic pain. Chronic-pain patients expect the worst. They go through life waiting for the other shoe to drop.[11] The tendency to make things out to be worse than they are is called catastrophizing and is the strongest determinant of the tendency to develop chronic pain.[12] The stronger the catastrophizing, the more severe the pain.[13] Catastrophizing is also part of depressive thinking.

FAMILY MATTERS

The pain-depression complex is a family affair. Social forces are also at work, which is why it is helpful for chronic-pain teams to include a social worker. Chronic pain impacts family members. Their reactions affect how the person with pain copes with it. Some families have a positive influence, others more negative. Among married couples, this depends upon whether the relationship has been strong and supportive or full of anger, tension, fighting, and criticism.[14]

Look at Georgette and Burt. They'd had a good marriage, but it wasn't perfect. Georgette lived with bottled-up disappointment and resentment over Burt's lack of attention. Chronic pain now gave her Burt's undivided attention. The more Georgette suffered, the more attention she got. Yes, she paid a terrible price for Burt's attention, but people are complicated.

Family members of my patients with chronic pain sometimes tell me they feel their relative is doing it for attention. Let's be clear. There are much better, and less unpleasant, ways to get attention. And I did not find Georgette to be a conniving sort. Actually, I've never seen a chronic-pain patient whom I thought was. Georgette was miserable and would have been overjoyed to be rid of the pain. I thought that depression explained the severity of her pain. It also made her feel helpless and dependent, and this made her receptive to Burt's hovering.

Chronic pain often gets twisted up in complicated family relationships. When this happens, family therapy (counseling) may help the entire family cope more successfully with the elder's pain and lessen its impact on all involved. Pain may not get better until depression is effectively treated and family matters are addressed.

TREATING THE PAIN-DEPRESSION COMPLEX

Among patients with both chronic pain and depression, treatment of depression improves both depression and pain.[15] Treatments widely used for depression can be effective for chronic pain. In fact, they work for chronic pain even when depression is not present. This may be further evidence that chronic pain and depression involve overlapping brain functions and makes antidepressant treatment a good choice for treating the pain-depression complex.

We have known for many years that antidepressant medications can help with chronic pain. In recent years, the Food and Drug Administration has approved certain newer antidepressant medications for the treatment of pain. But others work as well. Serotonin norepinephrine reuptake inhibitors (SNRIs) and tricyclic antidepressants (TCAs) are used the most, but others may be as effective. When SNRIs or TCAs cannot be used, it may be worth trying members of other groups of antidepressants.

Psychotherapy, a mainstay treatment for depression, can also help with chronic pain. One form of psychotherapy, cognitive behavioral therapy, may be especially effective. In this treatment, therapists work with patients to identify patterns of depressive thinking and to understand their connection to chronic pain. This can help patients learn not to catastrophize.[16]

"SHRINKING" CHRONIC PAIN

If you are struggling with chronic pain, or you have a relative who is, when should you think about seeking the help of a mental health specialist, such as a psychiatrist? As I've indicated earlier, it's never a bad idea and ought to be part of any thorough chronic-pain team evaluation. But often it's not. So, if a mental health specialist is not already involved, here are some indications to get one involved:

- Severe emotional distress is part of the overall picture.
- One or more treatments for the pain fail to work as expected.
- The pain causes more disability than expected from the cause of the pain.
- The person demands more pain medicine than ought to be needed.
- The person wants ever-increasing doses of narcotic pain medication.
- Depression is present, especially prior to surgery for the pain.
- Pain seems associated with behavior problems or symptoms.

- The person with chronic pain has suicidal thoughts or behaves in a self-destructive manner.

THE BAD NEWS

Chronic pain can be tough to control. Once the pain-depression complex sets in, it gets tougher. Some patients do not get better. I do not know what became of Georgette, but I wasn't able to make her better.

I treated Georgette with a number of different antidepressant medications. Several didn't agree with her, but others did. Unfortunately, they didn't relieve either her depression or her pain. I also got Georgette and Burt to come for marital therapy. But this didn't do much good either, and after three sessions they dropped out and never returned.

CONCLUSION

Chronic pain is a very common problem for older adults. Older adults with chronic pain too often do not receive adequate treatment for it, especially if they also have depression. Family members have an important role in making sure that their older relative gets good treatment for both problems.

There are two common errors to watch out for. The first is that depression goes unrecognized, gets ignored, or is inadequately treated. If someone you care about has depression, then, before they receive powerful narcotic pain medications or undergo pain injections, nerve blocks, or surgery, they ought to have treatment for depression. It might be the best ticket to feeling better and might spare them one or more medical procedures.

The second problem is inadequate treatment of pain. Sometimes older adults with severe depression do not receive adequate attention for their pain. Making sure their pain is properly addressed is equally important.

16

DON'T TAKE THE FALL FOR DEPRESSION: DEPRESSION AND FALLING

About one-third of older adults living at home, and half of those living in nursing homes, fall each year. Half of these individuals fall multiple times.[1] One-fifth will be injured, and half of these will be very serious.

Falls can be catastrophic and life changing for older adults. Broken bones and internal injuries may require surgery, and painful and prolonged rehabilitation may be needed. Some older patients never fully recover from a fall, their lives changed forever. In the aftermath of a fall, some older adults who had been living at home will be forced to enter long-term care facilities.

Even when physical injuries heal completely, and function returns, falls can be psychologically traumatic and leave deep, emotional scars, which can be just as crippling. Insecurity, self-doubt, anxiety, and depression take hold and can be hard to shake off. It should not be surprising that falling can trigger depression. But depression also causes falls.

WHY OLDER PEOPLE FALL

Falling is associated with frailty in older adults. But no simple, single reason explains why older adults fall. Falling is one of the geriatric syndromes. You may recall that geriatric syndromes are complicated health problems that do not have a single cause. They often arise when multiple functions break down. Incontinence is another geriatric syndrome.

Risk factors explain why depression and falls are often seen together. A wide range of abnormalities can contribute to falling. Muscle weakness, impaired mobility, poor balance, posture problems, and cognitive impairment are often part of the picture. Cardiac disease, cerebrovascular disease, arthritis, Parkinson's disease, and diabetes are common root causes. The illnesses and disabilities that lead to falls also cause depression. Smoking, drinking, and inactivity also increase the chance of falling.[2] And a wide range of medications, prescribed for many types of health problems, can be a factor.

When it comes to cognitive impairment, it is the executive functions that cause trouble with falls. Other forms of cognitive impairment, including memory disorders, are not a problem.[3] We reviewed the executive functions in chapter 4. These are the command-and-control abilities that are important for paying attention to the environment, concentrating on what you are doing, anticipating hazards, and making the necessary adjustments. Most of the time we take these for granted. But I think you can easily appreciate how important these functions are, operating behind the scenes, for any of us not to trip, stumble, and fall.

So when trying to understand why a particular elderly person has fallen, many possible reasons must be considered. Depression is one more.

CAN YOU REALLY FALL FROM DEPRESSION?

Yes, you can. Many studies link depression to falls. Some researchers estimate that older adults with depression have 50 to 60 percent more falls.[4] The more severe the depression, the more frequent are the falls.[5] This relationship may represent a vicious cycle. Falls trigger depression, which brings on more falls, and so on. Around it goes, each problem making the other worse, a pattern we have seen with several other conditions.

HOW DOES DEPRESSION MAKE YOU FALL?

We do not really know how depression causes falls. It probably does so in a number of ways. As I alluded to earlier, some effects may be indirect. Depression increases the chance of other problems that lead to falls, such as cerebrovascular disease, drinking, and inactivity. The physical inactivity of depression can very quickly decondition the muscles of older adults. As we have seen already, individuals with depression often do not take medications correctly. This has been shown to be associated with falling.

Depression also causes the depression-executive dysfunction syndrome. As I described earlier, persons with impaired executive functions are easily distracted and don't pay close enough attention to their footing. This leads to falls. And the brain circuits affected in depression are also linked to motor function and mobility. This may explain why older adults with depression have more difficulty walking. They take shorter strides and have longer periods with their weight on both feet than is normal,[6] and this may lead to falling, too.

MYRNA

Myrna had been depressed for ten years when I met her. The prolonged depression had taken a toll. She was in tough shape, and she was only seventy-two.

Myrna's depression had been unrelenting, although not for lack of trying to treat her. She'd been hospitalized for treatment four times, with absolutely no improvement. Umpteen different medications for depression, in various combinations, had been tried, by a succession of psychiatrists. Because nothing made her better, several of her doctors had recommended electroconvulsive therapy (ECT), often known as shock treatment, but Myrna wouldn't agree to have it.

Ted, her husband, was dead set against ECT and wouldn't allow it. He brought Myrna to me, hoping that a geriatric specialist might be able to succeed where all the others had failed.

Myrna and Ted had both been teachers. They had been enjoying an early retirement filled with tennis, golf, and dancing, until Myrna's depression struck. Ted was still athletic and robust, but ten years of depression turned Myrna into a frail old lady who looked ten years older than her age.

When I met Myrna, she looked haggard. She hunched over, shuffled along, and seemed to move in slow motion. Her face was drawn, and her expression was downcast. She was fretful, worried, pessimistic, sad, and anxious. Her thinking was rigid and inflexible, and she catastrophized about everything. She'd had diabetes for a few years but hadn't taken very good care of it and had tingling in her feet from diabetic neuropathy. Myrna had already fallen once, and, since then, she had been hesitant to leave her home.

Myrna had treatment-resistant major depressive disorder. Ten years of it had left her fairly disabled. She had muscular weakness and walked like a frail little old lady. And she'd fallen once already. I did not like the idea of treating Myrna with more medication. Good treatment with medication had already failed many times. Neither tricyclic antidepressants nor monoamine oxidase inhibitor antidepressants had been tried. While these medications sometimes work better, I was very worried they would substantially increase her chance of falling. Instead I recommended ECT or another nonmedication treatment called transcranial magnetic stimulation (more about all these treatment options in later chapters).

Myrna didn't want any part of shock treatment or transcranial magnetic stimulation. Ted had been sure I would offer more medication treatment, and Myrna had set her hopes on this. Despite my concerns about the low chances of success and the substantial risks, they implored me to treat, and I did. In hindsight, I'm not sure I would do the same thing again.

The first thing I tried was adding an antipsychotic medication to Myrna's antidepressant regimen. This seemed the least risky and offered some hope of success. Myrna did get a little better but not much, and the new medication made her walking slower and less steady. I took her off it. Next I tried gradually replacing one of her antidepressants with a tricyclic antidepressant. This helped her sleep better, and she thought it reduced the tingling from her neuropathy, but it also made her lightheaded and wobbly, and she fell.

Fortunately, Myrna was not injured, but the fall was nevertheless traumatic. Myrna became more anxious and afraid of falling. At her next appointment, Ted told me she'd become afraid of the stairs, saw herself as too frail to get in and out of the car without help, and had confined herself to four rooms of their home, where she felt more confident on her feet. Ted led her into my office, holding her by the arm. Her feet seemed to not want to move, as if they were magnetized to the floor. Each step was an effort. She needed help to sit down and stand up. She was weaker and more disabled.

In the interim, Myrna had been to a neurologist who could find no physical reason to explain why her walking was so impaired. The neurologist concluded that anxiety was the culprit and recommended renewed efforts to treat it. Obviously he did not know all the details of Myrna's treatment.

I again recommended ECT, but Myrna declined. I also thought any further treatment ought to take place in the hospital, but both Myrna and Ted had had enough of these places. Wasn't there anything else we could try? A very low dose of lithium was one last thing that had never been tried. Sometimes it helps antidepressant medications work, and I agreed to try this one last thing.

Unfortunately, on the way home, Myrna fell on her driveway and broke her collarbone and wrist. She spent three days in the hospital and then went to a rehabilitation facility. Sadly, she made no progress, and her walking became even weaker. After four futile weeks, she went to a nursing home for long-term care, and I never saw her again.

FEAR OF FALLING

What transformed Myrna from a tennis-playing, youthful retiree to a feeble old woman? In hindsight, depression was probably primarily responsible. Early on it made her withdrawn and inactive, and she quickly fell out of shape and gradually weakened. Later, depression kept her from managing her diabetes, and she developed neuropathy in her feet, which added to her unsteadiness. Had she stayed active and in shape, maybe she wouldn't have developed diabetes at all. Her first fall made her insecure, and the second one was more unnerving and left her with severe fear of falling.

Fear of falling refers to anxiety about falling that seems excessive or leads to unnecessary restriction of activity. It is normal for older adults living at home to worry about falling. Such concern usually reflects a realistic desire to adjust to aging and is not fear of falling. Steps elders can take, including improving nighttime lighting, removing clutter and obstructions in their homes, and wearing more stable footwear, make common sense and prevent many falls.

I cannot say enough about proper footwear, so I hope you will indulge a brief story about this. I once treated an eighty-seven-year-old former beauty queen who was falling once or twice a week. She would not trade in her high heels for rubber-soled walking shoes. "Wear old-lady shoes, no way!" she told me emphatically. She couldn't see the connection between her falls and her footwear. Vanity was part of it, but the real problem was poor executive cognitive functions, which left her without a suitable level of anxiety about falling.

Fear of falling is often triggered by a fall. Even minor falls can be demoralizing and emotionally traumatic for some older people. Fear of falling can also arise for no apparent reason. Even though fear of falling is a form of anxiety, depression appears to be a much stronger trigger.[7] The more severe the depression and the more intense the fear of falling, the greater the activity restriction will be.[8] Once fear of falling sets in, it can trigger a downward spiral of activity restriction, social isolation, increased anxiety and depression, weakness, and more falls. Permanent disability may be the result.[9] This was Myrna's fate.

FALLS AND ANTIDEPRESSANT MEDICATIONS: BALANCING RISKS

Myrna's decline was pretty dismal, and I was not able to help her. We'll never know whether things could have turned out better if she had had the ECT. Depression is treatable, and the vast majority of older adults can avoid fates such as Myrna's without needing ECT. Most get good results with antidepressant medications.

But there is a dilemma: while depression increases the risk for falling, so do antidepressant medications. Various kinds of medications increase the risk of falling. Antidepressants are among them. Not all studies confirm that antidepressants increase falls. But it is generally accepted that they do, and you may have read or heard this elsewhere.

So if you have depression, is it safe to take antidepressant medications? The simple answer is yes, if you need them. If you have already had one fall, then depression increases your chance of falling again, more so than taking antidepressant medication does. The scale tips in favor of taking antidepressant medications, in general. But everyone is different, so you need to work with your doctors to decide what is best for you.

Doing nothing is not a good choice, unless you are prepared to follow Myrna's path. It's not that she did nothing, but she didn't make the best choices open to her (more on this in a minute). But what choices do you have? Do you need antidepressant medications?

Psychotherapy can be as effective as medication for all but the most severe depression. It even works sometimes for fear of falling.[10] One advantage of psychotherapy is that it does not have the side effects of medications. Myrna was not interested in psychotherapy. She'd had a lot of it during her ten-year odyssey of depression and saw it as useless. To be fair, in the condition she was in, I didn't think it would help her.

I was also not optimistic about medications. A very large number had already failed. A few stones had been left unturned, but these options had very high risks of causing falls, and the odds of success seemed low. Nevertheless, Myrna and Ted wanted to press on with medication, and I respected their preference.

I would have preferred that Myrna have ECT. Had she agreed to ECT years earlier, she might have spared herself the decline that drove her into a nursing home. Who knows, she might have even recovered substantially and been able to play tennis again—she might have gotten her life back!

We will cover ECT in detail in chapter 22. For now, suffice it to say that ECT is more effective than medication, often works even when medication has failed repeatedly, and avoids the side effects of medication.

FALLS AND DEPRESSION: DON'T MISS YOUR CHANCE TO PREVENT BOTH

Falls can be an emotionally traumatic experience that triggers depression, and depression increases the chance of falling. When both are present, as was the case with Myrna, a vicious cycle and downward spiral can occur.

Myrna's story is grim, but it doesn't have to be for you. The good news is that prevention is possible, and I think this is a reason to feel hopeful.

Exercise and tai chi can prevent both falls and fear of falling.[11] Participating in these activities helps older adults feel more confident on their feet. Successful treatment of depression improves not only emotional well-being but also the executive functions needed to avoid falls. Treating depression thus reduces the risk of falls and lessens your chance of many other health problems.

Part III

How to Beat Depression to Stay Healthier and Live Longer

17

"YOU CAN LEAD A HORSE TO WATER . . ."

Getting a Reluctant Elder to Accept Treatment

Irma was eighty-nine. She came to see me with her husband, Dick, and daughter, Patricia. It was Patricia who had called to make the appointment, which she had advised the office staff was "for Irma's depression." When I ushered Irma into my office, she was polite, cooperative, and pleasant. So far, so good. But Irma wasted no time in letting me know that she had been brought in "under duress." She saw no reason to see me. It had been "their idea" (Dick and Patricia's), and Irma disavowed any knowledge of the reason.

Many of my first encounters with patients start this way because seeing a "shrink" for depression is usually not their idea. More often than not, "traitorous" family members have instigated it, sometimes at the primary care physician's behest (treachery knows no bounds). Despite their distrust over being brought to a psychiatrist, older patients are usually polite and respectful. This generation was raised to put on fresh underwear before going to the doctor. Even those who come in shooting daggers tend to be on their best behavior.

Of course, not everyone is. I've had patients storm out of my office in a fit of rage. Others cooperate with family members only as far as my office parking lot. Once there, they refuse to get out of the car. Not knowing what to do, their family members come into the office to explain the situation. Mostly they seem embarrassed by their uncooperative family member or ready to blow their stacks over his or her behavior.

When this happens, which happily is not too often, I have two patients on my hands: the one refusing to get out of the car and the one melting down in my reception area. The receptionist sits the family members down with a cup of coffee while I try to see the patient in their car. When I knock on their car door window and introduce myself, they are so flabbergasted that they let me in.

People do some interesting things in the back of automobiles, but psychiatric treatment ordinarily is not one of them. But half the time I manage to convince my would-be patient to come into the office. And many of those who refuse to budge eventually return and willingly come into the office.

What magic do I work on these tough customers? There's no secret to it. Older adults usually find me to be a nice guy who is easy to talk to. Once they see I am listening to them and seem to understand and respect their feelings, they want to talk to me.

Treating older adults for depression often requires first convincing them to do something they do not want to do. I start the doctor-patient relationship off on a good note by meeting them where they are. Sometimes this literally means in their car. Other times it means making a house call. House calls are often not feasible, but they can be an effective way to break the ice with geriatric patients who will not go to the office. I find that house calls disarm defensive elders by reminding them fondly of their younger years, when the practice was commonplace.

Even when the first encounter is a conventional office visit, as it was with Irma, much patience is needed. It takes time to understand older adults' doubts about treatment of depression and to allay their concerns. They cannot be rushed. If you understand this, you'll be in a better position to help ease the reservations of an older adult you care about.

Rather than focus initially on Irma's depression, I tried to get to know her as a person. She wanted to talk about her family, even though she had been unhappy with them a moment earlier. She and Dick had been married sixty-four years. They'd had a good marriage. He'd been a loyal and loving husband. Patricia was the most rock-solid and dependable of her four children. She was devoted to her parents and would do anything for them. This made it hard to understand such a "betrayal." Irma suspected that "they think I'm crazy." Worse yet, she feared that "they want to have me put away."

Irma was mortified and scared. I empathized with how upsetting it is to be ganged up on by family members and be dragged off to a strange doctor, a psychiatrist, no less. I acknowledged that she seemed to be in an uncomfortable predicament, but I told Irma it puzzled me. What on earth would make such trusted family members behave in such a way? Initially Irma claimed she had no idea, but in time she admitted that her "memory was shot." Maybe they were worried about her because of that. Maybe they meant well but were misguided. Then she admitted that she too was worried about her memory, and it seemed to be getting worse.

Now we were getting somewhere. Irma had revealed a concern, and I followed her lead. I again held off asking her about depression and instead showed concern about her memory problems. I asked her to tell me her biggest worries about it. Immediately Irma revealed she was afraid of not being able to take care of herself. She didn't want to be a burden on her family, feared not being able to recognize them, and dreaded spending her last days living in a "snake pit" strapped into a chair in a drugged-up state.

I told Irma this sounded terribly bleak to me, and she sounded gloomy and hopeless. She said this "summed it up pretty good." She felt down in the dumps all the time and worried constantly. She had been expecting the men in the white coats to come to take her away any day and had assumed I would order this. Rather than endure such a fate, she had considered doing away with herself but didn't know a painless method. Anyway, she reassured me that suicide was against her religion, and she didn't want to do anything to hurt her family. I guess she didn't really feel they were traitors after all.

I told Irma I thought I could help her and asked whether she would be interested in treatment. She looked uneasy and said she wasn't sure. So I quickly observed how nice it had been to meet her, gave her my card, and invited her to return any time that she decided she could use my help—no hard sell. Then I got up to usher her out of my office, but Irma was not ready to leave.

As if she were doing me a favor, Irma said she would come for a second visit. She also allowed me to talk to Dick and Patricia about their concerns. It doesn't always go this smoothly. Getting over this first hurdle is often more challenging. But once older patients see for themselves that the geriatric psychiatrist is a supportive professional who understands their problems, they are usually glad they came.

Here's what Dick and Patricia told me. Irma had been a smoker and had high blood pressure but had been well until a heart attack four years earlier. A flurry of small strokes followed. After the dust settled, she was not as sharp as she had been and was somewhat depressed. Then driving became a problem. A string of moving violations and minor fender benders forced Dick to forbid her to drive. This had been his first "traitorous" act and had hurt terribly. Thereafter depression steadily worsened. For three months prior to seeing me, she had been eating poorly and was losing weight; she sat on the living room sofa all day with the shades drawn, just staring into space.

Dick and Patricia seemed like reasonable people, and they were obviously very worried about Irma. But they had run out of patience and were clearly disappointed in me that I let Irma leave with nothing more than another appointment. Patricia looked as though she wanted to grab Irma by the shoulders and shake some sense into her. Irma's "stubbornness" was hard for her to take. The patience required during this time often seems too much for many family members to bear, but bear it they must. Sometimes the surest path to treatment is quite roundabout. Depression caregivers need as much help as do those for Alzheimer's patients, maybe more. This is one reason I consider late-life depression to be a family illness.

Irma very much wanted to feel better, but she could not bring herself to fully consent to treatment. It took several visits before Irma at last agreed to try medication for depression. She kept finding additional reasons to decline a prescription for an antidepressant. First she clung to the denial about having depression. Then she was afraid to take "mind-altering," addicting medications that would put her in a fog. I allayed each concern in turn, but she found new reservations. Next came criticism that doctors, me included, just "pile on more and more pills." Then there were worries about the side effects and safety of antidepressant medications. At each visit I made sure Irma understood that treatment was up to her. And once she started, she could stop at any time.

Between visits, Dick and Patricia "worked on" Irma to convince her that she had nothing to lose by letting me treat her for depression. Their efforts, though well meaning, made my job more difficult. They increased Irma's worry that I was on her family's side, not hers. The problem, you see, is that Irma, like many older adults, feared she had a lot to lose.

As older adults become frail and sense their independence slipping away, they begin to fear losing control of their lives. Nothing brings this out more than the suggestion that they have a mental health problem or need psychiatric treatment. The current generation of older adults grew up in a time when mental health problems were causes of shame and embarrassment. They were taught that the "proper" approach to emotional problems was to keep them secret and deal with them privately. Psychiatric treatment carried an enormous stigma and often meant confinement in an "asylum." In my experience, the more older adults feel pushed into treatment, the more tenaciously they resist it. The negativity and pessimism that are part and parcel of depression just add to the problem.

What do you do when faced with such a dilemma? Dick and Patricia got Irma to see me, but what if you are not having much luck getting even that far with an elder you feel very worried about? What can you do? Here are some dos and don'ts to keep in mind.

- Do try to see past what appears to be stubbornness in order to understand the person's point of view.
- Do assume an older adult with depression has reasons for rejecting treatment that feel very rational to him or her. In other words, try to understand what it might mean for the older adult to acknowledge the need for treatment—that they are weak, "crazy," helpless, and so forth.
- Do take these reasons seriously, and try to find out what they are.
- Do listen sympathetically and avoid contradicting or negating his or her feelings.
- Do accept older adults' feelings as valid, even when they seem irrational to you.
- Don't try to talk them out of how they feel, or try to talk sense into them.

- Steer clear of too forcefully trying to get them to listen to reason. This may backfire by convincing them that you really do not understand them.
- Do accept the terms older adults prefer. Irma would have no part of treatment for depression but was interested in help to feel less down in the dumps. Older adults who adamantly deny they have depression may readily admit that they feel low, down, or miserable.
- Don't expect to persuade older adults to seek professional help for depression without first convincing them that you understand their concerns and take them to heart.
- Do back off and try again when the timing is better, unless the situation is dire.
- Don't give up; too much is at stake.

Not until the fourth visit to my office did Irma accept a prescription for an antidepressant. It was already three weeks since Irma's first appointment, and two months since her family had made that appointment. It felt slow as molasses to Dick and Patricia, but at last we were getting somewhere . . . we thought. Two days later, Irma's daughter called to tell me that Irma had not yet started taking the pills. She was still "thinking it over." In frustration, Patricia wanted to put Irma on the phone for me to "lay down the law" with her. It doesn't work this way. Patricia didn't want to hear that I thought it would be better to respect Irma's concerns and address them face-to-face at her next appointment. I thought flames were going to shoot out of the phone. But, absent urgent situations, patience, which Dick and Patricia were out of, remains the surest route.

Medical treatment of any kind rarely succeeds when patients do not accept it is in their interest to have it. Treatment in these situations either doesn't work well or actually backfires. Older depressed patients often need additional time to accept the idea that taking medication for depression is a good idea. Few patients have as much doubt and hesitation as Irma, but most have at least some. Irma did finally start taking her medication, but already a month had passed. This delay had not gotten us off to a running start, and I did not yet know it would take ten months for her to get better (spoiler alert for chapter 21).

POSSIBLE WAYS TO EASE ELDERS' DOUBTS AND HESITATIONS

Now that you have the general idea, let's get more specific. I won't say I've seen it all, but after more than thirty years of practice I've seen a lot—lots and lots of depressed older adults with various reasons for declining treatment of depression. Every older adult is unique, but I've noticed common patterns in my patients' objections. In the remainder of this chapter, I'll describe these objections and suggest approaches you can try to help an older adult feel comfortable accepting treatment.

Objection 1, Denial: "I Do Not Have Depression"

Many older adults would rather have leprosy than admit to having depression. Blame stigma and false beliefs about depression and psychiatry, which we covered in chapter 1, for this ingrained obstacle. And ingrained it is.

Suggested Approach

I have said enough about this already in the list of dos and don'ts. Remember, what you call it makes no difference as long as something is done about it.

Objection 2, Denial: "My Problem Is Not Depression; It's Pain!"

Or trouble breathing, a churning stomach, or fatigue . . . you name it. Depression causes a wide range of physical complaints. Because of the stigma associated with mental health problems, many older adults find it more palatable to focus on physical problems and deny the presence of depression, even when it's the cause. Depression can cause physical complaints, and it can make physical problems worse.

Suggested Approach

It usually does no good to challenge older adults' views of their problems. So don't do it! And for goodness' sake, don't say anything that even implies you think their physical problems are all in their head. It may only make them more defensive.

Recognize the physical complaints as real. They are, in one sense or another. If an older adult says his or her problem is trouble breathing, then it is, whether the cause is emphysema or depression. Older adults may be more open to hearing that stress or emotional factors are making their physical symptoms worse. Explained in these terms, older adults might accept that treatment for "stress," "nerves," or even "depression" is necessary to relieve their physical complaints.

Objection 3, Denial: "I Can't Be Depressed Because I Have No Reason to Be Depressed"

This rationalization relies on the belief that depression is a normal reaction to depressing events rather than a brain disease.

Suggested Approach

I find helping older adults understand that depression is a brain disease goes a long way. You may find it helpful to reread chapter 2. Some older adults with depression may not have the energy or motivation to read the entire book but might be able to read that chapter. I reassure my patients, "It's not you; it's your brain . . . it's let you down."

Objection 4: "I Don't Need Help; I Can Handle It Myself"

You may remember my patient Don, from chapter 1. He rejected medication for depression because he couldn't accept the idea that he wasn't "sailing his own boat." The pills he took for his thyroid, heart, and lungs were okay because "you have no control over those organs." But he saw medical treatment for the mind as different because "you should be able to control it yourself." Such thinking is often behind patients' steadfast insistence that they must pull themselves out of it.

Suggested Approach

This is a tough barrier to break through. My relationship with Don was such that I could challenge his stance, using his own metaphor, by pointing out that his boat seemed to be sinking and I was worried he was about to go down with the ship. This would not have been suitable for most patients. Most often the best approach to try first is to point out, as gently as you can, how they are not functioning and thus not handling the depression themselves. If this doesn't sway them, try turning to information from any of the chapters in part 2. In my experience, handle-it-yourself stoicism sometimes gives way when patients learn that depression is not a harmless condition but one with potentially devastating effects on health and longevity.

Objection 5: "Forget It! I'm Not Crazy!"

You might be surprised how often older adults with depression fear that others think they are losing their minds, going crazy, or becoming senile. They act as if admitting having depression or accepting help for it is the first step to being "put away."

Suggested Approach

In the gentlest, most nonthreatening voice you can muster, explain that you are puzzled about what makes them so opposed to treatment that would help them. Then ask the depressed elder whether he or she has been afraid of being thought crazy and in need of being put away. Reassurance and facts go a long way. I explain that depression is a mood disorder caused by failure of emotion circuits in the brain, which sometimes become unbalanced with aging or stress. I reassure them that it has nothing to do with being crazy, losing their minds, or going senile. Their relief is so great that you'd think they'd been told by an oncologist "it's benign; you don't have cancer."

Objection 6: Peer Pressure

Older adults sometimes have difficulty maintaining their privacy. I see many residents of senior housing, retirement communities, and assisted-living facilities. Believe me, the gossip mills in these settings can be vicious. Older adults, being mindful of the stigma of mental illness, worry about being labeled and ostracized. If word gets out, there will be no shortage of well-meaning friends and neighbors offering advice. Some is positive: I receive a number of word-of-mouth referrals from my success-story patients. But peers often cast a negative pall over treatment of depression.[1]

Suggested Approach

This is a very real, practical problem for many older adults, and I sympathize about it. I remind my patients that their problems are no one else's business and advise them to do what they must to make sure it stays that way. I suggest that this may be one of those times that call for little white lies.

Objection 7: Fear of Psychiatry

Psychiatry has come a long way since the time of Freud and the mental asylums. Nowadays, a visit to a geriatric psychiatrist more closely resembles a trip to the family doctor than a session with the archetypal stern, silent, bearded psychoanalyst. However, geriatric psychiatrists usually have more time than most primary care physicians and are easier to talk to. Nevertheless, older adults fear psychiatry as coercive.[2] Frail older adults, who feel their independence slipping away, often fear they will be forced to reveal personal secrets, take medications against their will, or be locked up in a mental ward.

Suggested Approach

At least once a week, new patients comment that their visit with me was nothing like they imagined—it was much better. I suggest telling older adults that seeing a psychiatrist is not what they think it is. They can go once and see for themselves. If it is awful, they do not have to go back. It will be their choice.

Objection 8: Admitting Needing Help for Depression Is the First Step into the Nursing Home

No one gets "put away" for depression, but it's amazing how many older adults believe this still happens.

Suggested Approach

This is a very real fear that needs to be taken seriously. Don't dismiss it as ridiculous. Here are two facts: No one gets put in a nursing home for depression. Some people are put in nursing homes due to the disabilities that depression can cause. I suggest telling older adults that ignoring depression is not the way to stay out of a nursing home; having treatment for it is. As far as the problem of needing a nursing home goes, treatment for depression is not the problem; it's the solution.

Objection 9: "They'll Just Pile on More Pills"

Older patients take a lot of medications. They come to expect that any visit to the doctor with any complaint will result in more pills. You would be surprised how often my patients confide in me that they purposely didn't tell their other doctors about a serious symptom to avoid more pills.

Suggested Approach

First, it's easy to understand older adults' feelings about this. In general, the older you are, the more medications you need. This is a lousy aspect of aging, and every time more pills are added, it gets lousier. But what's the alternative? Would those with depression really be better off spending the rest of their lives depressed, getting sicker and sicker, and dying prematurely? Earlier I advised against trying to drum sense into the heads of depressed elders. But when depression robs older adults of their common sense, family members may need to help them think this through sensibly. Often, healthcare decisions involve choosing the least bad choice.

Here's a ray of hope you can offer. We know that many older adults actually do take more medications than is good for them. Geriatric specialists try to figure out which medications might be harmful or unnecessary and can be stopped. Geriatric psychiatrists are familiar with those that can cause depression, and it is not unusual for geriatric psychiatrists to recommend that one or more medications be stopped. So it is reasonable to encourage older adults to see a geriatric psychiatrist by holding out the possibility of fewer medications, not more.

Objection 10: Fear of Side Effects

Dire warnings about the side effects of medications are everywhere: pharmacists hand out lists with prescriptions, television commercials for new medications mention them, and then there's the Internet. Fear of side effects is legitimate. Bad things do happen. But depressive thinking causes many older adults to blow side effects out of proportion. Many of my patients think side effects are inescapable rather than the rare occurrence they are. I am also surprised how often my patients believe they will have to remain on medications that cause serious or troublesome side effects.

Suggested Approach

Death and taxes are a sure thing, not side effects. Start with reassurance that the Food and Drug Administration (FDA) does not approve medications that cause side effects 100 percent of the time. I also go to great lengths to reassure my patients that antidepressant medications are intended to help them feel better, not make them feel worse. These medications are not addicting, so we can lower the dose or stop them right away if they cause unpleasant or intolerable side effects.

Objection 11: Fear of Being "Doped Up"

Older adults worry about this a lot. Many assume that medications psychiatrists prescribe are "mind-altering drugs" that will turn them into doped-up zombies.

Suggested Approach

Reassurance that antidepressant medications should make depressed individuals feel back to normal and not doped up may help. Medications that make patients feels worse are not doing what they are supposed to do and should be stopped. Agreeing to try a medication is not a lifetime commitment. It's a day at a time.

Objection 12: "I Don't Want to Get Addicted"

Older patients often assume that all psychiatric medications are addicting. I see many depressed older adults who have received prescriptions from their well-meaning primary care physicians for tranquilizers such as alprazolam (Xanax), lorazepam (Ativan), and clonazepam (Klonopin). These sedatives are prescribed to hold patients over until they see me. I have always been struck by the irony of patients expressing reservations to me about the antidepressants I recommend being addicting, yet they do not know the tranquilizers their primary care doctors prescribed for them are highly addicting. And they never asked their primary care doctors!

Suggested Approach

Fear of addiction is a form of fear of losing control and must be addressed. I go out of my way to make sure my patients know that antidepressant medications are not addicting, because many are uncomfortable asking.

Objection 13: "I Don't Want to Be Experimented On"

Medications for depression take a long time to work, and there is no guarantee they will. Patients find the possibility of having to start over very disheartening. I don't blame them. There's no way around it; it is a trial-and-error process. Older adults sometimes view this as experimentation, and they object to being treated as guinea pigs.

Suggested Approach

There is nothing experimental about antidepressant treatment. Medications not yet on the market, being testing in clinical trials, are experimental. Antidepressants already available for doctors to prescribe are fully approved by the FDA because they are scientifically proven to work. There is nothing experimental about them. Treatment of depression is not an exact science. It requires clinical judgment, and there is a trial-and-error aspect to some of it. But this is also true of treatment of many other illnesses, including arthritis, high blood pressure, Parkinson's disease, epilepsy, and elevated cholesterol.

Objection 14: "I Don't Want to Talk About It"

Older adults grew up during the heyday of the Freudian era. Many still assume that seeing a mental health specialist for depression involves this type of treatment, and they fear it. They were raised to keep emotional problems to themselves and not to air dirty laundry, especially personal feelings. They imagine that psychiatrists have ways of making patients reveal all kinds of embarrassing or shameful secrets.

The best-intentioned family members can unwittingly play into this reservation. As I have pointed out in prior chapters, relatives sometimes firmly believe that their loved one is depressed over some deep-seated psychological problem. They feel hopeful that psychiatrists can "drag" these hidden conflicts out of their relatives and, in so doing, relieve their relatives' depression. The idea of having sensitive feelings dragged out of them by an intimidating doctor makes many older adults cringe. Any hint that this is in the offing just makes them circle the wagons even tighter. You can lead a horse to water, but you can't make it drink.

Suggested Approach

I advise family members of reluctant patients to tell them a few things about psychotherapy. Psychotherapy, commonly referred to as "counseling," is not the only form of treatment for depression. There are other types, which we will get to in the next chapter. Some older adults prefer psychotherapy to medications. Many do not. Older adults with depression have choices.

Second, most psychotherapy with older adults tends to focus more on finding better ways to handle current life challenges. It is more practical and tends not to delve into the past as much. And third, patients never have to talk about anything they are uncomfortable talking about. Once again, it's completely up to them.

IT IS NOT GULAG PSYCHIATRY

In the Soviet Union psychiatrists were co-opted by the state to control political dissidents. Fortunately this type of thing never went on in Western democracies and doesn't happen anymore in Russia. Yet, as we have seen, older adults fear that treatment of depression will subject them to strong-arm, coercive tactics. It is easy to see why. The perception of psychiatric treatment held by many persons who are old today harkens back to images depicted in the movie *One Flew Over the Cuckoo's Nest*. The psychiatric treatment portrayed in that classic film shares certain characteristics with Soviet gulags.

Loss of control late in life is a scary prospect, and loss of control of one's mind is scariest of all. It's easy to see why frail older adults fear being put away and link this with mental health problems. You probably noticed that much of my approach to elders' hesitancy about treatment for depression relies on reassurance, reassurance, and more reassurance. Irma certainly needed her share of this.

Admitting you have depression does not get you put away. The asylums have been closed, the men in the white coats are no more, and laws now fiercely protect individuals' rights to refuse treatment, especially psychiatric treatment. With enough reassurance that they will not be forced to have treatment they do not want, even the most negative older adults with depression become comfortable enough to give treatment of depression a try. They'll stick a tentative toe in the water.

Older adults' family members are often equally uncomfortable, albeit for different reasons. They feel worried and frustrated, and hope something at last will be done. As we saw with Dick and Patricia, having the patience needed is pretty tough. But there's no way around it. Older adults simply cannot be rushed into treatment for depression. They need time. Patience, more often than not, pays off, if the time is put to good use providing the reassurance older adults need.

18

YOU'RE NEVER TOO OLD

Treatments for Depression Work!

I've lost track of how many times I've made this point. Considering how debilitating depression is and the toll it takes on health and longevity, it is truly tragic that the vast majority of older adults with depression receive no treatment for it, when effective treatment is readily available.

We know that older adults with depression respond to treatment. Some respond as well as younger people but slower. Some patients get very good results. They get their lives back, stay healthier, and live longer. Maybe you will too. Others are not as fortunate. They respond poorly or not at all. But this is no reason to give up or forgo treatment completely. Quite the opposite. It's a reason to try harder.[1]

When I treat patients for depression, my goal is to help them get back to normal. I'm satisfied when they tell me they feel like themselves again. I wish I could say I achieve this with every patient. I don't—far from it. Geriatric treatment, of all kinds, often requires compromises. Sometimes perfect is the enemy of the good. I work closely with my patients and their family members to decide how good is good enough. I don't want to sell anyone short. Sometimes this means using all the tools in the toolbox to get the job done. In the remainder of this chapter, we'll review the tools for depression and get some idea about their place in treatment.

ANTIDEPRESSANT MEDICATION

I'm beginning with antidepressants but not because these are the most important. For better or worse, antidepressant medication is the treatment for depression most often used to treat older adults, that is, if they receive any treatment at all. For this reason, I've given antidepressant medications a later chapter of their own. For now, I just want to point out a few things that will give you a feel for the value of antidepressant medications as one of the tools in the toolbox.

Let's start by looking at what antidepressants are not. They are not "happy pills," "mood elevators," or "uppers," terms I hear people use. If antidepressants were truly happy pills, I suspect lots of people would take them recreationally and some would abuse them as they do illegal drugs. This is why we don't prescribe antidepressants for common forms of human unhappiness. Antidepressants treat illness. They work in major depressive disorder and other forms of severe depression, in which brain function is abnormal. In these conditions, antidepressants restore normal function through their chemical action in the brain.

How exactly do they do this? Antidepressant medications have numerous actions that impact the brain abnormalities in depression. They affect the monoamine neurotransmitters, alter gene expression, reduce inflammation, increase the release of brain-derived neurotrophic factor (BDNF), reduce oxidative damage, increase neuroplasticity, and promote sprouting of new brain cells in key areas related to emotions and memory.[2]

Wow! This is quite a list of impressive actions. It's likely that the other treatments described in this chapter, including psychotherapy, do much of the same. So where do antidepressants fit in? For mild to moderately severe depression, on average, antidepressant medications are no better than psychotherapy. In mild cases, complementary and integrative approaches may also help. But in severe depression, antidepressant medications work better than psychotherapy. Antidepressant medication combined with psychotherapy works the best, but if only one treatment is possible, medication is the right choice in severe cases.[3]

PSYCHOTHERAPY

Many older people do not understand psychotherapy very well. This treatment, sometimes known as the talking cure but more commonly referred to as counseling, intimidates some older adults. Others over-simplify psychotherapy as advice giving. Skeptics doubt the value of seeing a professional for what friends, family members, or the local bartender will give them for free.

One thing psychotherapy is not is advice giving. Bartenders, lawyers, accountants, stockbrokers, plumbers, decorators, friends, and family members all give advice. Even doctors give advice about their patients' health. I certainly do. Good psychotherapists don't give you advice about living your life. They cannot know what advice is right, because people are too complicated. Instead, psychotherapists help people to understand themselves better so they can feel better about themselves and make the best decisions possible for themselves.

So what is psychotherapy? One characteristic involves work. Like physical therapy, you have to put in effort to make progress. And like physical therapy, the adage "no pain, no gain" often applies. Psycho-therapy is not always enjoyable. Sometimes you find yourself talking about things that are unpleasant or even emotionally painful.

This aspect contributes to the stigma of psychotherapy. Some people fear somehow they'll be made to talk about deep, dark secrets they do not wish to discuss. Nothing could be further from reality. Psychothera-py is a partnership between therapist and patient. Therapists are not mind readers, and no therapist can force anyone to talk about anything they wish not to bring up. It is always up to the patient.

Older adults often assume psychotherapy involves lying on a couch. On entering my office for the first time, patients often ask, "Where's your couch?" It puts their minds at ease when I tell them that very few psychiatrists still do that kind of treatment, and I never had a couch. Most psychotherapy with older adults, these days, is done sitting up in a chair and focuses on current life problems, what makes them hard to cope with, and better ways to handle them.

Healthcare professionals widely assume that older people prefer medication to psychotherapy, and this is often true. Many members of today's older generation were raised not to talk about problems. They tend to see mental health problems as a form of personal weakness or failure. Taking a pill often feels more acceptable to them. Some research suggests this is not always the case; some older people would rather have psychotherapy and avoid pills.[4] Unfortunately, not enough people feel this way. Psychotherapy works as well as medication for milder depression, and it does so without the side effects that medications can cause.

Just as there are different types of medication, there are different forms of psychotherapy. In the past, long-term treatment was common and went on for years. Short-term treatment, typically ten to twenty visits, is more standard now. Let's get a basic feeling for the different forms of psychotherapy.

Cognitive behavioral therapy is based on working with patterns of depressive thinking or acting. The therapist helps the patient to identify repetitive patterns of thinking or behaving that are negative, pessimistic, and self-defeating, and result in bad feelings, such as depression or anxiety. Interpersonal psychotherapy identifies changes or conflicts in relationships, such as grief or role transitions, that cause bad feelings. Psychodynamic psychotherapy identifies how problems in the past may affect experience in the present. It is similar to psychoanalysis but is much less intense or in-depth. Reminiscence therapy involves reviewing aspects of one's past in order to see oneself in a new light. And problem-solving therapy involves learning new strategies to deal with current problems more successfully.

Psychotherapy is particularly helpful when mental health problems occur in connection with various life stresses or crises. Some of the more common stresses or difficulties in the lives of older people include grief, loss of independence, loss of an important or productive role in society or family, chronic illness, disability, chronic pain, moving to a new location, shifting relationships, coping with the diagnosis of Alzheimer's disease, being a caregiver, and facing death when it nears. The psychotherapy approaches described above can help people who may not be handling these challenges well to cope with them more successfully.

I have found that many older patients feel uneasy about trying psychotherapy. I encourage them to take the plunge, like getting into a pool of cold water. It may feel uncomfortable initially, and your first instinct may be to get out, but once you start swimming you warm up quickly and find it to be fairly pleasant. With psychotherapy, the first one or two sessions may feel odd or awkward. But if you keep at it, you may warm up, hit your stride, and find it to be pleasant at times and very rewarding. If not, you can quit any time. It's up to you.

Psychotherapy is not suitable for all older adults with depression. Many forms of psychotherapy depend on weekly sessions to work well. Transportation may not be available, or unpredictable health problems may cause frequent cancellations of sessions. Insurance may not cover the number of sessions needed, and out-of-pocket costs may be too much. Poor hearing, pain, bladder and bowel problems, breathing problems, and other physical symptoms may make it hard to pay attention during sessions. Poor memory may prevent progress from carrying over from one session to the next. And people with executive cognitive problems may no longer have the mental flexibility to see things in new ways or change their behavior.

It is not helpful to coerce an elder who does not want to have psychotherapy. Psychotherapy generally takes motivation and effort. You have to want to do it or, at the very least, not refuse it. The adage "you can lead a horse to water, but you can't make it drink" applies.

PHOTOTHERAPY

Phototherapy simply means using light for medical treatment. Dermatologists use light for psoriasis, acne, and eczema. Pediatricians use light for jaundice in newborns. Psychiatrists use light for certain types of depression.

Phototherapy works very well for seasonal affective disorder (SAD; covered in chapter 4). Some research shows it may help with other types of geriatric depression.[5]

How does light relieve depression? Daily bright light exposure keeps our twenty-four-hour biological clocks properly timed. Some of the body's twenty-four-hour rhythms are thrown off schedule in depression. Decreased exposure to natural light during the fall and winter months causes this in people with SAD. Phototherapy resynchronizes the body's twenty-four-hour rhythms, relieving the depression. To be effective, the light has to be perceived by the eyes. Bright light activates a sensor between the eyes and the brain, triggering reactions in the brain.

One nice thing about phototherapy is that you can do it right at home. But it's not without inconvenience. You have to sit in front of and look at a special light box early in the morning, thirty minutes to an hour per day, usually first thing in the morning. The light must have an intensity of ten thousand lux, which is a measure of brightness. To get a feel for this, bright, outdoor sunshine is about ten thousand lux of light.[6]

Phototherapy has effects in the brain similar to antidepressant medications. Treatment reduces the stress hormone cortisol and increases melatonin, the so-called sleep hormone, involved in timing the sleep cycle. Melatonin also improves mood and lessens anxiety.

In order to do phototherapy, you will need to buy a light box. These can be purchased in retail stores or online. The Food and Drug Administration does not regulate light boxes as medical devices, so be careful. Many of the light boxes on the market do not produce the type of light needed.

It is not a good idea to do phototherapy on your own. You ought to work with a psychiatrist with expertise in this treatment. Not only will you need guidance in buying the right kind of light box, but also you must have the right dose prescribed. Most important, before spending money on a light box, you need to make sure that light therapy is safe for you.

Phototherapy is safe for most patients. Patients with certain eye diseases, including macular degeneration or retinal damage from diabetes, should not use phototherapy. And patients who have no lens in an eye, after cataract surgery, should not have phototherapy.

No treatment, even psychotherapy, is completely without side effects and risks. Phototherapy occasionally causes nausea, dizziness, anxiety, restlessness, and headaches. If used by patients with bipolar depression, phototherapy can trigger mania.

Phototherapy is also not as tried and true for nonseasonal depression in the elderly as is antidepressant medication or psychotherapy. Compared with medication, it has the advantage of fewer side effects or drug interactions. And compared with psychotherapy it may be more convenient, although you need to do it daily. Phototherapy is a good option for many older adults with SAD who have the discipline needed for daily treatment. It may be an option for some older adults with other forms of mild depression. But it is often not practical for many older adults, especially those who are frail, disabled, or confused. In severe depression, turning to phototherapy instead of medication may delay other urgently needed treatment.

COMPLEMENTARY AND INTEGRATIVE APPROACHES

Mind and body practices, herbal treatments, and nutritional supplements are used to treat a range of health problems including depression. These approaches are collectively referred to as complementary and integrative health or complementary and alternative medicine. Many "natural" treatments are touted to work for depression. Some of them do and are useful additions to the toolbox. Others are unproven and may be useless. And not all natural products are as safe as people believe them to be.

I think it is reasonable for older adults to use complementary and integrative approaches for depression when there is at least some good scientific evidence that they work and are safe. Exercise, yoga, tai chi, Reiki, SAMe, omega-3 fatty acids, curcumin, and St. John's wort all fit this bill. There are two places for one or more of these treatments in the treatment of late-life depression. First, they can be tried, early on, instead of more conventional medical treatments, for mild depression. Again, in severe depression, it's a mistake to put all your eggs in this basket. You won't get better, and you'll be delaying treatment you're going to end up taking anyway. Complementary approaches can also be added to traditional medical treatments to make them more effective. More on all of this in a later chapter devoted entirely to these treatments.

ELECTROCONVULSIVE THERAPY

Yes, electroconvulsive therapy, often called shock treatment, and abbreviated ECT, is still used to treat depression, including depression in the elderly. In fact, ECT works better for severe depression in older adults than it does with younger people.

ECT is an extremely important treatment for a small number of patients who desperately need help. For this reason, and because there is so much misunderstanding and fear of ECT, I have included a separate chapter on it. For the moment, I simply want to make sure you understand ECT's place in the toolbox.

These days ECT is used infrequently. Antidepressant medications are effective enough that they have eliminated the need for ECT in most cases. This historical transformation in psychiatric treatment often seems lost on skeptics who believe that antidepressants are useless. ECT is reserved for patients who are seriously depressed and not getting better despite many attempts at treatment with medication and other therapies. In this sense, people often view it as a last resort. Very rarely, it is turned to sooner, when depression is so severe that it is life threatening.

ECT is faster and much more reliable than antidepressant medication. It is the most effective treatment known for depression. If you are trapped in a depressive illness that will not release its grip on you, ECT might be your ticket out.

TRANSCRANIAL MAGNETIC STIMULATION

We have seen that light can be used to treat depression. Transcranial magnetic stimulation, TMS for short, uses magnetism. TMS uses a highly directed magnetic field to stimulate areas of the brain affected in depression. Unlike ECT, patients remain fully awake during TMS. There are no intravenous injections or medications, as there are in ECT. Patients sit in a chair, much like a dentist chair, with a magnetic coil hovering just above their scalp. The treatment has no serious risks and is not invasive. Unlike ECT, which may be given up to three times a week for seven to ten treatments, TMS is given five days a week for four to six weeks. It is a much bigger time commitment but easier to undergo.

There has been some controversy regarding just how effective TMS is. Some studies show it to be as effective as ECT, but others raise doubt about this. Very few studies have been done with older adults. This is a huge limitation. From the data we have, TMS does seem less effective with older adults than younger people. It may be that the older you are, the less well TMS works.[7]

TMS is covered by Medicare but only if you already have tried two different antidepressant medications that didn't work. Patients continue to take their antidepressant medications during TMS. In this regard TMS is similar to ECT.

TMS is an option when antidepressant medications are not working. The jury is still out regarding whether TMS works as well as ECT, and trying more medication is just as reasonable. To have TMS you must be able to make daily treatments—you get weekends off—for four to six weeks. So if you can do this, and you either can't tolerate or do not want to try more medication, and are not ready to try ECT, TMS may be a good next step.

HOW DOES TREATMENT FOR DEPRESSION WORK?

Nobody knows exactly how the different treatments of depression work. Don't let this unnerve you or make you skeptical. The same can be said for lots of medical treatment. Lots of clinical research and sixty years of experience with some of these treatments bears out that they work.

While we do not know for sure how treatments for depression work, we have some pretty good ideas. During depression, some areas of the brain become underactive, others overactive, and the connections between brain areas malfunction. Treatment with medication, psychotherapy, or ECT corrects these abnormalities.[8] This is the key concept: depression is a disease caused by abnormal functioning of the brain; treatment, regardless of the type, works by restoring normal brain function. Imagine that! You can change how your brain works by talking with a psychotherapist.

USING THE RIGHT TOOL FOR THE JOB

So what is the right tool to treat depression? It depends on several factors. These include the type of depression you have, how severe it is, how long you have had it, your past history, your preferences about treatment, and the availability of certain treatments in your area.

If you have mild depression and want to do something about it but are not inclined to take medication, and psychotherapy does not appeal to you, you might start with complementary and integrative approaches. You could do this on your own, or work with a holistic healer, but I think this is unwise. You need to get a thorough checkup with your primary care doctor first to make sure something else is not causing your depression. And I think you will be better off seeking out a medical specialist who uses these approaches.

If instead you prefer more mainstream treatment, you might start with psychotherapy. Medication remains an option, but bear in mind that not all psychiatrists believe that medication should be prescribed for milder forms of depression.

Now let's say you have a more severe depression. It drags you down, day in and day out, is hard to shake off, and makes it hard to function. You should approach this as a serious medical illness. Be prepared to have psychotherapy or take medication. Combining medication and psychotherapy is the most effective thing you can do.

What happens if you do not start to improve within a few months? If you are in psychotherapy, you may need to consider adding antidepressant medication. If you are already taking an antidepressant medication, your primary care doctor should talk to you about switching to a different one. If you still do not improve, you should see a psychiatrist.

In chapter 23 we will examine what goes into good treatment, whether you are working with your primary care doctor or a specialist. For now, let's see what further steps are possible to get you moving down the path to getting better.

Further treatment with medication might include switching to a different type of antidepressant, combining two or more antidepressants, or augmenting your antidepressant with other types of medications. Augmentation involves adding different types of medications to antidepressants to make them more effective. Lithium, thyroid hormones, psychostimulants such as methylphenidate (Ritalin), and antipsychotic medications are among the medications that sometimes help antidepressants do their job better. If you are not already using complementary and integrative approaches, adding one or more might also be an option.

Still no improvement? Does it feel as if you've tried every medication in the pharmacy? Don't give up hope. This is the time to start thinking about TMS or ECT. I usually recommend ECT, but for patients who want to avoid it at all cost, TMS is an option. If TMS fails, you can still have ECT. I know that the prospect of ECT makes many readers uncomfortable, but try to think of it as a safety net, if all else fails.

ONCE YOU'RE WELL

You finally feel better. What a relief! I've had patients tell me they had forgotten what it felt like to feel like themselves. One patient joyously described to me all the activities she had resumed. She was trying to catch up for lost time and get reacquainted with herself. Imagine that. Now that you feel great, is it okay to stop your medication? No, no, no, no, no! That's the last thing you want to do.

Just because you feel good doesn't mean the depression is gone. It's no different than diabetes or high blood pressure. If you stop treatment the problem comes right back. In fact, your improvement is a fragile state. Once better, older adults who have been treated for depression are more prone to relapse.[9] Again, this is not a reason to sit on the sidelines. It's a reason to stay in the "game" and apply the "full-court press" to defend against the return of depression. A rule of thumb in geriatric psychiatry is "the treatment that makes you better is the one you should stay on." Older adults who stay on their medication for depression and continue to have monthly psychotherapy sessions, even once they feel fine, have half the relapse rate over a three-year period.[10] Stick-to-it determination is needed.

CONCLUSION: A WORD TO THE WISE

In this chapter I have distilled down to bare bones information about the range of treatment for late-life depression that is available as I write the book. Scientific understanding of depression is improving rapidly, and more and better treatments are on the horizon. Depression is a complicated illness, and older adults are all unique. Treatment that is right for one might not be for another, even if they appear to share many similarities. Please use this information to ask your doctors questions so they can work with you to find the treatment that is most right for you.

19

WHEN LIFE GIVES YOU LEMONS, MAKE LEMONADE

Antidepressant Medications

If you have depression you really need to do something to get rid of it. I sincerely hope that you agree and that your only remaining question is which type of treatment is best. In this chapter, we will take a closer look at antidepressant medications.

For better or for worse, antidepressant medications are the treatment for depression older adults are most likely to receive. This is not always a good thing. But if you have severe depression, then antidepressants are probably your best bet.

Unfortunately, antidepressant medications are not perfect—far from it. True, the choices currently available work great some of the time. I have patients who praise their antidepressant as a "miracle." Usually antidepressants are less than miraculous. They take a long time to work and often do not work as well as we hope. At least half the time the first one tried does not work at all.[1] Multiple attempts with different antidepressants are often needed. And antidepressants have side effects. Sometimes side effects necessitate abandoning one antidepressant and starting over with another.

Because of these limitations, it is easy for patients and their family members to get discouraged. This is entirely understandable, but don't give up! If you know what to expect, stick with treatment, and work closely with your doctor; then more often than not you'll get better. If you know more about antidepressants, you can ask better questions, make smarter decisions, and receive more effective treatment.

WHY DO WE USE ANTIDEPRESSANT MEDICATIONS?

"Can't you just give me something for nerves, like Xanax?" is a question patients or family members often ask me after I recommend an antidepressant medication. They fear antidepressants as powerful psychiatric medications with serious side effects. In contrast, they are at ease with Xanax and the other Valium-like tranquilizers called benzodiazepines (doctors like to call these benzos, for short, and so will we), viewing them as mild and harmless. They couldn't be more mistaken.

In my experience, many people don't realize there are different types of psychiatric illness, each involving different brain circuits and having a specific treatment. They see mental health problems as a common result of not being able to cope and treatment as easing "bad nerves." In their minds, the important differences between psychiatric medications is whether they are mild or strong: "everyday pills," such as Xanax, which many people seem to take, or powerful "psychotropic medications" with a stigma attached to their use.

An even more important difference is that patients feel benzos working within minutes, but antidepressants can take weeks or longer. When you are sick, you want something that makes you feel better quickly. Take an antidepressant and nothing happens, except maybe side effects. Take a benzo and you feel calmer right away. Common sense tells you one works and the other is useless. You have to understand a lot about the treatment of your disease to stick with the antidepressant.

Sure, benzodiazepines will make you calmer and more relaxed in the short term, but they will not relieve your depression. Long-term, they might make it worse.

This is no different than having bacterial pneumonia. Tylenol will reduce the fever, and oxygen will ease your breathing. Both do this within minutes. But if you do not take antibiotics you will not get better. You might even die! We use antidepressant medications and not benzodiazepines for depression for the same reasons that we use diabetes medications and not asthma medications for diabetes.

People with depression need a treatment that does more than help them feel less upset. They need treatment that corrects the malfunction of the brain circuits affected in depression. Antidepressants do that.

HOW DO "HAPPY PILLS" MAKE YOU HAPPY?

Let's start by recalling what antidepressants are not. As I said in chapter 18, they are not "happy pills," "mood elevators," "uppers," or "mood lifters," terms my patients often use.

So what exactly do antidepressants do in the brain? They alter levels of monoamine neurotransmitters. They cause changes in gene expression, which affect the regulation of key proteins. They change the function of brain cells and circuits they make up. And they reduce inflammation and oxidative damage, and increase brain-derived neurotrophic factor (BDNF). One result of all this, maybe the key result, is that neuroplasticity, the sprouting of new brain cells and the formation of billions of new connections, improves and the brain gradually resumes normal operations.[2]

ALL ANTIDEPRESSANTS ARE NOT ALIKE

Once patients agree to take an antidepressant, they still ask me, "Can you give me a mild one?" It's a sensible request. You don't take a powerful narcotic pain reliever for back pain before first trying a milder pain reliever such as Tylenol or Motrin. Unlike pain medications, though, there are no strong or weak antidepressants. All are equally effective, with two exceptions we'll come to. In this regard they are all similar.

In other aspects, antidepressants are different, and there are a few families that many of them belong to. These families include the selective serotonin reuptake inhibitors (SSRIs), serotonin norepinephrine reuptake inhibitors (SNRIs), tricyclic antidepressants (TCAs), and monoamine oxidase inhibitors (MAOIs). Several antidepressants do not fit in any family. Regardless of where they belong, all antidepressant medications treat depression. What distinguishes them is the slightly different ways they work to accomplish this.

Even within a single family, antidepressant medications may have subtle differences in how they work and big differences in their side effects. So, whenever you see a one-size-fits-all description of antidepressant side effects and risks, it's probably an oversimplification. Let's review the different antidepressants so that you will have at least some idea of the different groups and how they differ. I'll go through them in order according to how commonly they tend to be prescribed for older adults, from most common to least.

Selective Serotonin Reuptake Inhibitors (SSRIs)

You may recall that serotonin is a monoamine neurotransmitter. The others are norepinephrine (also called noradrenaline) and dopamine. Neurotransmitters are released by one nerve cell to communicate a message to another nerve cell. This is how information is conveyed from cell to cell in brain circuits.

As the name implies, SSRIs affect serotonin. After serotonin has been released, SSRIs prevent brain cells from taking it back up. The released serotonin lingers longer between cells, amplifying the cell-to-cell message.

Common SSRIs include fluoxetine (Prozac), sertraline (Zoloft), paroxetine (Paxil), citalopram (Celexa), and escitalopram (Lexapro). The lowercased names are the generics. Fluoxetine works great, but geriatric psychiatrists tend not to use it. It is extremely long acting, which means it builds up, takes a long time to clear out of the body, and has a lot of drug interactions. These characteristics can spell trouble for older adults. Paroxetine is also not ideal. It has moderate anticholinergic side effects (I'll explain these later), something geriatric psychiatrists try to shield their patients from.

SSRIs can cause upset stomach, loose bowels, and insomnia, but they are generally freer of side effects than other groups. For this reason, SSRIs are the antidepressants most doctors turn to first.

Serotonin Norepinephrine Reuptake Inhibitors (SNRIs)

This group includes venlafaxine (Effexor), duloxetine (Cymbalta), and desvenlafaxine (Pristiq). These medications are broader spectrum than SSRIs: in addition to blocking the reuptake of serotonin, as SSRIs do, the SNRI medications also block the reuptake of norepinephrine—they do more. When an SSRI does not work, one option is to switch to an SNRI in hopes that it will work better because of its additional action in the brain. SNRIs cause similar side effects to SSRIs, but they are more likely to cause headaches, nausea, and sweating.

Mirtazapine

Mirtazapine (Remeron) is a noradrenergic and specific serotonergic antidepressant and is in a class by itself. It works on serotonin and norepinephrine (noradrenaline) but in a different way. When SSRIs and SNRIs fail, mirtazapine may succeed. Mirtazapine also stimulates appetite and induces sleep, and it's a pretty good treatment for nausea. It can be useful when depression is accompanied by loss of appetite and insomnia. Mirtazapine is sedating and makes some older adults logy. It can also cause lightheadedness and dizziness.

Bupropion

Bupropion (Wellbutrin) is also in a class by itself. We do not know with certainty how it works, but it may affect dopamine and parts of the brain affected by nicotine. Bupropion does not cause weight gain, sexual side effects, or sedation, so it may be a good choice when these are a concern.

Vilazodone

Vilazodone (Viibryd) is a newer antidepressant that has SSRI action and also helps with anxiety. Older adults tolerate it well.

Vortioxetine

Vortioxetine (Brintellix) is a newer and different type of antidepressant. It is a serotonin modulator and stimulator. Vortioxetine has SSRI activity, but it has complex effects on other serotonin systems. It may also be worth trying when other antidepressants have not helped.

Tricyclic Antidepressants

The tricyclic antidepressants (TCAs) are one of the oldest families of antidepressants. Older adults who had depression earlier in their lives may be familiar with some of the common members, which include amitriptyline (Elavil), doxepin (Sinequan), imipramine (Tofranil), nortriptyline (Pamelor), and desipramine (Norpramin). In very severe depression, TCAs may be more effective than other families, an important difference. Unfortunately, TCAs also have more side effects. They must be used with great caution, and some older adults should not take them.

Heightened concerns about TCAs come from their anticholinergic (see below), sedating, blood-pressure-lowering, and cardiac side effects. Amitriptyline and doxepin are very strongly anticholinergic and are not usually recommended for geriatric use, although they can be helpful under certain circumstances. TCAs should be monitored with electrocardiograms to ensure they remain safe for the heart. And they should not be given to individuals recovering from a heart attack. One advantage of TCAs is that their levels can be measured by a blood test. This helps doctors adjust the dose to the right amount.

Monoamine Oxidase Inhibitors

The monoamine oxidase inhibitors (MAOIs) may also be familiar to older adults who had depression when they were much younger. The MAOIs are the oldest family of antidepressants and include tranylcypromine (Parnate), phenelzine (Nardil), isocarboxazid (Marplan), and one newer agent, selegiline (Emsam). The MAOIs are very effective. In fact they are more effective than TCAs. Unfortunately, they are also the most difficult for people to take. MAOIs have many side effects, including weight gain and lightheadedness, and patients must follow a special diet to avoid the "cheese effect." The cheese effect is a severe, possibly life-threatening rise in blood pressure that occurs when MAOIs interact with a chemical, called tyramine, found in certain foods, most notably— you guessed it—cheese. MAOIs are rarely used any longer because of the dietary restrictions and their many side effects. But they often work better than other antidepressants, and specialists familiar with their use still turn to them for patients who respond to nothing else.

Miscellaneous Medications with Antidepressant Action

Some of the antipsychotic medications are approved for bipolar depression. These medications are rarely prescribed alone for other forms of depression, but they may used to augment antidepressants (see "What Next," below).

Psychostimulants, such as methylphenidate (Ritalin) and combinations of amphetamine and dextroamphetamine (Adderall), are familiar treatments for attention deficit disorder. They have a fifty-year track record for geriatric depression. You may occasionally see them used for this purpose, either alone or to augment more conventional antidepressants.

ANTICHOLINERGIC SIDE EFFECTS

Now that I have used this long word several times, let me tell you what it means. Many different types of medications have anticholinergic side effects. These side effects include dry mouth (if you think it is difficult to pronounce "anticholinergic," try saying it with a dry mouth), constipation, difficulty starting the urine stream, and blurry vision. When severe, anticholinergic side effects can cause urinary retention or bowel obstruction.

While these side effects are very serious, even more worrisome is the memory impairment and confusion that anticholinergic medications can cause. Anticholinergic medications block the action of the neurotransmitter acetylcholine, the main neurotransmitter for memory and other cognitive abilities. This effect can cause forgetfulness, a picture that mimics Alzheimer's disease, and delirium. I think you can see why we try to avoid anticholinergic medications when possible.

Paroxetine and mirtazapine are somewhat anticholinergic, and amitriptyline and doxepin are highly anticholinergic. These medications can still be used as long as an individual is not taking additional anticholinergic medications. Bladder medications such as oxybutynin (Ditropan) and tolterodine (Detrol) are anticholinergic. So are ranitidine (Zantac) and cimetidine (Tagamet), two medications to reduce stomach acid. There are many others. Usually it is the additive effect that gets people in trouble. This is why it is so important for doctors to monitor all of their patients' medications and consider this list when prescribing any new treatment.

HOW DO PHYSICIANS DECIDE WHICH ANTIDEPRESSANT TO USE?

As I mentioned before, all things being equal, most doctors will turn to SSRIs first. If the first one does not work, they may even try a second one.

If a patient has severe insomnia and poor appetite with weight loss, mirtazapine might be a good choice because it can rapidly improve sleep and appetite. Because older adults take a lot of medications, it's always an advantage when an antidepressant "kills two birds with one stone." On the other hand, mirtazapine might be a poor choice for an overweight individual with diabetes. Bupropion has no cardiovascular or sexual side effects, does not cause weight gain, can help people quit smoking, and sometimes improves energy and ambition, so it can be a good choice when these issues are important. In general, medications that are shorter acting and have fewer possible drug interactions are good choices, and those that are anticholinergic, sedating, or cause lightheadedness are less ideal.

WHAT NEXT?

What happens when the first, second, or even third antidepressant does not work? Unfortunately, this is a real possibility. The good news is that there are many options. I find that my older patients take comfort in hearing this. Too often older patients expect doctors to give up on them, so I reassure them that I will stick with them as long as they want to stick with me.

After two or three attempts at treatment fail, each new attempt at treatment has only about a one in four chance of working. But more often than not, eventually a combination turns out to be a winner. It's like having a key ring with thirty keys on it. If you try them one by one, you'll probably find the one that unlocks the door. But you could end up locked out holding a lot of useless keys.

So, what are the next steps? The choices come down to switching, combining, or augmenting. Switching means replacing the antidepressants that failed with another of a type not yet tried. The rationale is that a medication that works differently might work better. It might be the key that fits your lock. Typically an SSRI is switched to an SNRI, bupropion, or mirtazapine.

Combining means taking two or more medications that all work differently to create a broader spectrum treatment. SSRIs plus bupropion or SNRIs plus mirtazapine are examples of commonly used combinations.

Augmentation is the practice of adding a different type of medication to an antidepressant. Antipsychotic medications, lithium, methylphenidate, and thyroid hormones are used to augment antidepressants. Finally, when none of these approaches works, doctors might turn to TCAs or MAOIs and start the process all over again.

How do doctors choose among so many options? Foremost, it must be case by case. Each patient's overall health and the list of medications he or she already takes must be considered. From this doctors can decide which side effects and drug interactions pose the greatest concern, and pick medications to avoid these. Patients' convenience and preferences, and the drugs' costs, must also be considered.

COMMON MISUNDERSTANDINGS

Antidepressants are complicated. They are much misunderstood. Over the years, I have been impressed by the amount of incorrect information floating around, particularly regarding use of antidepressants by older adults. Let's try to clear up some misunderstandings.

Old People Don't Get Better

We know this is plain wrong. We covered this in chapter 18. Enough said.

Antidepressant Medications Are Not Any Better Than Psychotherapy or Placebos

This is partially true. Antidepressants make the most difference and work better than psychotherapy in severe depression. No discussion! If you have psychotic depression or bipolar depression, there's no doubt—you must take medication or you are unlikely to get better. But in milder depression, psychotherapy is as good as medication and may be a better choice.

Antidepressants Make Old People Suicidal

Plain wrong! Antidepressants can increase suicidal feelings in teenagers and young adults, but this is controversial. There is no controversy with the elderly. Antidepressants reduce suicidal feelings among older adults.[3]

"I Don't Want to Be Hooked"

One dimension of stigma in psychiatry is the belief that all psychiatric medications are addicting. Narcotic pain medications and benzos are addicting. Antidepressants are not.

Patients sometimes ask, "If the medication makes me feel better, and then I stop taking it and I feel worse, doesn't that mean I'm dependent on it?" Well, yes. But that's no different from diabetes, arthritis, or breathing medications, which help people feel better. If a medication, including an antidepressant, makes your life better, you keep taking it. That's not addiction.

"I Don't Want to Take Mind-Altering Drugs"

Another concern is that antidepressant medications are mind-altering drugs. No, depression is mind altering. Antidepressants are mind restoring; they help make you you again. By the way, benzos can be mind altering. That's why they are abused and antidepressants are not.

Antidepressants Are Not Safe for Patients with Heart Disease

We covered this in chapter 6. To recap, the gist of it is that depression is not safe for your heart; antidepressants, for the most part, are safe. When it comes to heart disease, these medications are not part of the problem; they're part of the solution.

One exception is the SSRI citalopram. Citalopram is a popular medication for the treatment of geriatric depression because it has few side effects, is fairly short acting, and has few drug interactions. Under certain conditions, citalopram can cause a risky alteration in the heart's electrical rhythm called QT prolongation. When severe, this condition can lead to cardiac arrest and sudden death. Yikes! Fortunately, the risk is low as long as the dose is not too high, you take no other medications that also cause QT prolongation, and potassium is not low. With proper medical precautions, citalopram is safe to use.

Antidepressants Turn Patients into Drugged-Up Zombies

True, some antidepressants are sedating, and patients may feel drowsy, foggy, and out of it after taking them. This is an unwanted effect and usually a reason to abandon a medication and try something different. Most antidepressants do not do this. To the contrary, many must be taken in the morning because they cause insomnia if taken too close to bedtime.

KEEPING SIDE EFFECTS IN PERSPECTIVE

Side effects must be taken seriously. Dealing with them is job number one. Before we can wonder about whether an antidepressant will work, we need to know whether side effects are a big problem. If side effects are present, are they manageable? Can we adjust the medication to lessen the side effects? If not, the medication will have to be stopped, and we'll have to try again with another antidepressant.

You ought to be concerned about side effects. Bad things can happen. But try not to blow the risks of antidepressants out of proportion. The list of side effects you see for any medication is frightening, but they are not a sure thing; you are not guaranteed to get them. To the contrary, side effects are usually infrequent. And many side effects are nuisances and annoying but usually not dangerous. Others, such as falling, can be dangerous. But depression is dangerous too.

In my experience, excessive worry about antidepressant side effects reflects stigma and fear of psychiatry. Many of my patients fret about antidepressants yet accept far more toxic, risky treatments from other specialists for physical problems without flinching. Adverse effects from medication cause one hundred thousand hospitalizations per year.[4] Yet antidepressants do not make the list of the top six responsible drugs.[5]

Do antidepressants have risks? Sure they do. But let's keep it in perspective. Driving, going up and down the stairs in your home, and eating the food on your table all have risks. You make decisions to bear those risks every day for obvious reasons. Antidepressant risks must be weighed against the risks of depression, including all the possible ways it can ruin your health and shorten your life.

Now that we have that out of the way, let's look at some of the more common and concerning side effects of antidepressants.

Falls and Fractures

Antidepressants are associated with an increased rate of falling. TCAs and MAOIs are especially prone to cause falls. They lower blood pressure, causing older adults to become lightheaded when they stand up. SSRIs and SNRIs tend not to cause lightheadedness, yet they still increase the risk of falling, possibly by affecting balance.

As we saw in chapter 16, depression also increases the risk of falling. So you need to weigh the risk of falling from depression with the risk from antidepressants.

SSRIs pose another risk related to falls. They can reduce bone mineral density, possibly worsening osteoporosis and increasing the risk of fractures. Does this mean you shouldn't take SSRIs if you are worried about osteoporosis? No, it doesn't, especially if an SSRI is the best choice for you for other reasons. But if you already have decreased bone mineral density or difficulty walking, you and your family ought to keep a close eye on your walking to make sure you are not getting more wobbly. You should also see your doctor about treatment for osteoporosis and physical therapy to improve your mobility and strengthen your walking.

Other Side Effects

SSRI antidepressants increase the risk of bleeding very slightly. The risk is trivial for most people. But if you are on an SSRI and having frequent nosebleeds, the SSRI might be the cause. And if you happen to be dealing with a bleeding problem, it may be best to take a different type of antidepressant. People taking warfarin or other anticoagulants may also be at higher risk. SSRIs very rarely cause low sodium. And just as seldom, they cause an abnormally slow heart rate. Mirtazapine can cause a drop in white blood cells, so this should be monitored from time to time. Bupropion increases the risk of seizures, but the rate is very low, just 0.3 percent, so this is not a concern unless you are prone to seizures.

GIVE THE DEVIL HIS DUE

Ask yourself this: are any of the possible side effects that you might get from an antidepressant, but probably won't, really worse than the misery the depression causes you and the risks to your health that you now know about? Antidepressant medications are not perfect, but for now they are what we have. They might be lemons, but we can make pretty good lemonade with them.

Antidepressant medications work well more often than not. It's easy to focus on the failures and horror stories you hear and lose sight of how many people get better. One in ten Americans takes antidepressant medications. That's a lot of people, and most of them have good results.

20

LIFESTYLE PRACTICES, HERBAL TREATMENTS, AND NUTRITIONAL SUPPLEMENTS

Do you take glucosamine and chondroitin sulfate for arthritis? What about ginkgo biloba for your memory, fish oil for your heart, or saw palmetto for your prostate? Have you tried acupuncture for pain or started exercising to lower your blood pressure? If you answered yes to any of these questions, then you are one of the many millions of people using complementary and integrative health, CIH for short.

You might be surprised to learn that at least 40 percent, and maybe as many as 50 to 60 percent, of older adults use a variety of integrative therapies.[1] In fact, they do so more than younger people and have made integrative therapies a multibillion-dollar industry in the United States. CIH includes herbal therapies, probiotics, nutritional supplements, treatments such as acupuncture, and mind or body practices such as meditation.

I have included a chapter on CIH for three reasons. First, there is some evidence that some CIH therapies might have beneficial effects in depression. Second, many of my patients ask about CIH approaches for depression, so I assume that older adults everywhere are interested. And, finally, those older adults with depression who are inclined to use CIH ought to know something about it for depression.

COMPLEMENTARY, ALTERNATIVE, OR INTEGRATIVE HEALTH?

The National Institute of Health now refers to these nontraditional treatments as complementary and integrative health. There are many definitions of "integrative" health care, but all involve bringing conventional medical treatment and complementary approaches together in a coordinated way.[2] You may see CIH referred to as complementary and alternative medicine or simply integrative medicine. The name complementary and integrative health is coming into fashion as more and more of these practices are being used side by side with conventional medical treatment. As they become mainstream, they are less and less "alternative." And integrative "health" reflects the growing use of these approaches for health and wellness in addition to treatment of disease.

Most CIH approaches fall into one of two subgroups: natural products and mind and body practices. When I discuss treatment with my depressed patients, I include CIH among the options I cover. I recommend only those CIH approaches that we believe to be fairly safe and for which at least some evidence shows that they may help. The treatments we'll cover in this chapter fit this bill. They include omega-3 fatty acids, SAMe, folate, curcumin, St. John's wort, exercise, yoga, tai chi, acupuncture, and Reiki.

OMEGA-3 FATTY ACIDS (FISH OIL)

Fish oil contains omega-3 fatty acids and is good for your heart. The American Heart Association recommends that people eat fatty fish at least twice a week, and patients with coronary heart disease should take about 1,000 mg of the omega-3 fatty acids EPA and DHA daily. It turns out that omega-3 fatty acids are also good for your brain and may be helpful in depression. By themselves they may have mild antidepressant effects. But they may do more good when added to an antidepressant medication.[3]

Omega-3 fatty acids have a number of effects that may explain their depression-fighting actions. They reduce inflammation, increase brain blood flow, and improve the function of brain cell membranes. Omega-3 fatty acids also stimulate new connections between brain cells.[4]

The human body does not make omega-3 fatty acids, so we must get them from our diet. Fish and seafood are the best sources of omega-3 fatty acids. Walnuts and flaxseed are high in α-linoleic acid, which the body can convert to omega-3 fatty acids, so these are also good dietary sources.

Omega-3 fatty acids are safe for the majority of older adults. Cases of bleeding have been reported in association with omega-3 fatty acids, but there is no evidence that this is a common problem, and most people can take them without concern. In my experience, at least 3,000 to 4,000 mg per day, divided into three portions, is needed. I rarely recommend more, just to be on the safe side. People taking anticoagulants (medications such as Coumadin or Plavix) or using more than 3,000 mg of fish oil must do so under the supervision of a physician.

CURCUMIN (TURMERIC)

Turmeric is an Indian spice used in Ayurvedic and traditional Chinese herbal medicine to treat many conditions. In traditional Chinese medicine, it has been used for centuries to treat depression. Curcumin, a plant polyphenol, is believed to be the medicinal ingredient of turmeric. But does it actually work?

There is scientific evidence that turmeric has antioxidant and anti-inflammatory actions. Studies show that turmeric has some benefit for the treatment of osteoarthritis and inflammatory bowel diseases, such as Crohn's disease and ulcerative colitis, and it may also have cancer-fighting actions.[5] In the test tube, curcumin has been shown to fight brain inflammation and to prevent buildup of amyloid, the toxic protein in Alzheimer's disease. And turmeric does have some antidepressant effects.[6] No studies on turmeric for depression have included elderly patients, so we do not know whether it is helpful for late-life depression.

Side effects of curcumin include diarrhea, rash, headache, and yellow-colored stools. Blood clotting may be slowed somewhat, so patients taking warfarin (Coumadin) or other blood-thinning agents should use turmeric with caution, and it is prudent to stop taking it a few weeks before having surgery.

Despite the lack of proof that turmeric helps older adults with depression, some patients with depression may nevertheless wish to try it.

Not all patients respond well to standard approaches such as antidepressant medication or psychotherapy. Adding curcumin to these treatments seems reasonable. Those with very strong preferences for integrative approaches instead of standard medical treatments may wish to try curcumin before turning to prescription medications, as long as their symptoms are mild.

If you decide to try curcumin for depression, how much should you take? We don't know for sure. Five hundred milligrams per day is probably not enough,[7] but 500 mg twice a day may do the job, so this is a good place to start.[8] Curcumin is not absorbed well from the intestines and penetrates the brain poorly. It is believed that piperine (brand name BioPerine), an ingredient found in black pepper, improves the absorption substantially. Therefore, it may be best to use a curcumin product that also contains piperine or BioPerine.

SAME

The dietary supplement s-adenosyl methionine, SAMe for short, has been used to treat depression in European countries for decades. By itself SAMe can be effective some of the time for depression in adults.[9] SAMe may be a good alternative to prescription medication for some older people with mild depression, but it may do more good added to antidepressants.[10]

SAMe is a naturally occurring substance, made mostly by the liver, and found throughout the body, including the brain. SAMe works with folic acid and vitamin B_{12} in the manufacture of monoamine neurotransmitters. Some people with depression have low levels of SAMe. Dietary supplements may correct this deficiency and thus provide relief for depression.

The effective dose of SAMe appears to be 400 to 800 mg twice daily. Because we do not have research on the use of SAMe in older people, it may be prudent for older adults to start with 200 mg once or twice a day and increase the amount slowly. SAMe appears to be well tolerated. Side effects are few but can include an increase in systolic blood pressure (the top number), upset stomach, or diarrhea.

FOLATE

Many patients with depression are deficient in the B vitamin folate, often known as folic acid. Depressed patients with low levels of folate respond more poorly to antidepressant medications. Adding folate can help.[11] Some depressed patients not yet on antidepressants respond to folic acid alone.

Folate is used in the nervous system to make SAMe, and this is an important step in the production of neurotransmitters. Folate deficiency thus limits neurotransmitter levels, a factor believed to be related to depression.

Taking folate supplements can conceal a vitamin B_{12} deficiency. Undetected B_{12} deficiency can lead to serious neurologic problems, so folate supplements should be used under medical supervision.

Some patients with depression have genes that make them unable to transport folic acid into their brains. For folate supplementation to help their depression, they must take a form of folate called L-methylfolate. L-methylfolate is regulated as a medical food (don't ask), which means you need a prescription to get it.

When should you consider folic acid supplementation, and how do you go about it? First, start with a medical checkup and ask your doctor to order blood tests to check your folate, B_{12}, and homocysteine levels. Homocysteine in a chemical involved in the B vitamin–SAMe production line. When it is elevated, folate is deficient. If you have depression and your levels of folic acid are low, or your homocysteine levels are high, taking folic acid supplements might help. If you take folate supplements, keep in mind that you might be one who needs to take L-methylfolate.

ST. JOHN'S WORT

St. John's wort is an herbal therapy that has been used to treat depression, particularly in Germany and other parts of Europe. Two ingredients of the herb, hypericin and quercetin, are believed to have antidepressant properties. St. John's wort has been touted to have actions similar to SSRI and MAOI antidepressants. In mild depression, St. John's wort may have helpful effects. The usual starting dose is 300 mg three times a day. Some studies use doses of 1,500 mg per day, or higher. In more severe depression there are no proven benefits. Side effects include headache and abdominal pain. St. John's wort can interact with a number of medications, so be careful and make sure your doctors know you are taking it. [12]

EXERCISE

Exercise definitely helps depression, although it is no panacea. [13] At best, exercise is moderately helpful; it cannot replace medical treatment for severe depression, but it may be worth trying in mild depression, and it can enhance the effectiveness of treatment of more severe depression. Some form of exercise can be part of every depressed patient's treatment. [14]

How does exercise help to reduce the symptoms of depression? One likely answer is that exercise increases levels of the protein brain-derived neurotrophic factor (BDNF), which we have come across in prior chapters. BDNF keeps the brain in good working order. Low levels of BDNF are associated with a number of mental health problems, including depression. Regular exercise raises BDNF levels, as do other treatments for depression.

In addition to its role in restoring brain BDNF levels, exercise also produces psychological benefits that counter depression. People who exercise regularly feel more self-reliant and self-confident, and they have an improved sense of well-being. These benefits lead to improved coping and better mood.

What kind of exercise is best? Both aerobic and strength training are helpful. A balance of both types may be best. Before adding exercise to your routine, see your primary care physician to make sure it is medically safe for you to exercise.

YOGA

Yoga is a five-thousand-year-old Indian spiritual tradition that is both a form of exercise and a type of mindfulness practice. Yogis, practitioners who subscribe to its benefits, believe that practicing yoga leads to harmony of mind and body and a quieting of the mind.[15] Yoga has become increasingly popular in Western countries. Many health clubs offer yoga classes, and elder services, such as senior centers and assisted living facilities, offer chair yoga for their frail, elderly participants.

Yoga is thought to reduce stress. It increases serotonin and dopamine in the brain and lowers cortisol levels. And yoga also increases gamma-aminobutyric acid, a neurotransmitter involved in anxiety and depression. So it makes sense that yoga might ease depression.

Many studies show that yoga helps with depression. Unfortunately, these studies are of variable scientific quality and include different types of depressed patients and many different styles of yoga, so it is hard to make too much of them or to be confident about how beneficial yoga truly is for depression.[16] Improperly doing yoga can cause injury, so it may be best to work with a qualified instructor.

TAI CHI

Originally developed as an ancient Chinese form of self-defense, tai chi is a stress-reducing activity that combines exercise and mindfulness practice. It is sometimes called meditation through movement. Tai chi is low impact and can be performed by many older adults.

Tai chi is touted as an excellent practice for reducing stress. It reduces inflammation levels in the body[17] and improves executive cognitive functions.[18] It may also relieve depression, particularly when used in conjunction with antidepressant medication.[19]

ACUPUNCTURE

Acupuncture involves the insertion of extremely thin needles through your skin at strategic points on your body. A key component of traditional Chinese medicine, acupuncture is most commonly used to treat pain.[20]

Traditional Chinese medicine explains acupuncture as a technique for balancing the flow of energy or life force—known as chi—that flows through pathways (meridians) in your body. Acupuncture practitioners believe that inserting needles into specific points along these meridians will rebalance your energy flow. Western practitioners take a more scientific view that acupuncture points are places to stimulate nerves, muscles, and connective tissue. Some hypothesize that this boosts your body's natural painkillers, modifies neurotransmitters, and reduces inflammation.[21]

There are over one hundred studies of acupuncture in depression, including geriatric depression and post-stroke depression. This is an impressive number, but they are not conclusive because of inconsistencies in how acupuncture was administered and how the research was designed.[22] So while there is reason to think that acupuncture might help, it is far from proven. We also do not know how effective acupuncture is, how it compares with other treatments, and how many treatment sessions are needed to get good results.

Despite these reservations, acupuncture is considered to be fairly safe. It may be worth adding to your depression treatment plan.

REIKI

According to the International Center for Reiki Training (http://www. reiki.org), Reiki is a Japanese technique for stress reduction and relaxation that also promotes healing.

Reiki is increasingly used in hospitals, hospice programs, and private-practice settings for a variety of illnesses and conditions. It has been touted for fibromyalgia, pain, cancer, and depression. A very limited number of studies show some benefit of Reiki in easing depressive symptoms.[23]

Practitioners of Reiki believe that a "life force energy" flows through us. High levels of this life force energy sustain health and well-being. Low levels are associated with unhappiness, stress, illness, and disease. Reiki practitioners also believe that life force energy can be transmitted from one individual to another via something known as the biofield. There is no proof that such things exist, and Reiki is best thought of as a spiritual practice. The Reiki healer places his or her hands in various positions on or over the recipient's body. Practitioners believe that this process transmits some of their life force energy to the person who needs healing.

There are no known side effects of Reiki. The only harmful effect of Reiki might result from relying on it for severe depression at the expense of delaying needed medical treatment.

COME CLEAN WITH YOUR DOCTORS

Studies show that older persons who use CIH usually don't tell their doctors.[24] They really ought to. Keep in mind that nutritional supplements and herbal therapies are medications, naturally occurring, but medications nonetheless. They work through chemical actions in the body, as do medications, so they can interact with prescription medications and have side effects. So always let your doctors know what CIH products you take.

Supplements and herbal therapies are also unregulated. Companies can claim benefits that are unsubstantiated. You can never be as confident of what's in the product as you can with prescription medications.

CONCLUSION

If you have very mild depression and you feel strongly about avoiding psychotherapy or taking antidepressant medications, it might be reasonable for you to try one or more of the CIH approaches we just reviewed. You can try them, as long as you are realistic. And you can add them to traditional medical treatments. If you take medication, for any reason, always let your doctors know what CIH products you take.

If you have severe depression, do not delay needed medical treatment by putting all your eggs in the CIH basket. You'll probably regret it sooner or later. And before starting any body practice, such as exercise, check with your primary care doctor, or cardiologist, if you have one, to find out what level of physical activity is safe for you.

21

THERE IS NO MAGIC PILL

Why Good Treatment Can Take So Long

It never fails. At least once a week a patient with depression, or a member of the patient's family, asks me, "You mean there's no magic pill?" The question comes out once it sinks in that the relief they hope for might take some time. The irony in their voices does not conceal the very real disappointment they feel. Sadly there are no "magic" pills or quick fixes for depression—yet. With the medications we currently have, treatment of depression can sometimes be a lengthy process. If you are dealing with depression, you probably do not want to hear this.

Maybe you've read that it takes three to four weeks for antidepressants to "kick in." Actually many older adults do respond that fast, and some even faster. Maybe you remember my patient Agnes, from chapter 1, who responded extremely well to an antidepressant.

Agnes was a ninety-year-old woman who had been forced to move into an assisted living facility after falling made it unsafe for her to remain at home. Agnes had moderately severe depression. She was sad and gloomy all the time, experienced no pleasure in living, felt worthless, and wanted to die. The first antidepressant Agnes tried quickly made her feel better. She took up painting, a hobby she'd given up after her children were born; began teaching art lessons to other residents; and became chairperson of the residents' council. You might recall that she told me, "This is the best time of my life. I'm enjoying myself in ways I never thought I could." Success! This is what I hope to accomplish every time I treat an older adult for depression.

Older adults with depression can respond to treatment as well as Agnes did. Many do. But sometimes it takes a lot longer, several months or more. No matter how long treatment takes to work, it always seems painfully longer than anyone wishes.

I wrote this book to encourage people with depression to get treatment. So why did I include a chapter emphasizing that treatment of depression can be a slow, drawn-out process? That's a strange way to inspire hope and an odd remedy for depressive pessimism. The reality is that, all too often, there is no quick fix for geriatric depression. I have found that when older adults know what to expect and are prepared for what could be a long slog, they feel less hopeless when they don't get better right away and more hopeful that eventually they will get better.

Patience pays off. If you have depression, you need to muster all you can, stick with treatment, and not give up. If you are a caregiver, you must also remain patient and realistic. Unavoidable snags in treatment may come along, but there are things you can do to keep the process moving forward. Keep in mind that, with good treatment, the majority of older adults with depression get better.

Remember my very hesitant patient, Irma? We met her in chapter 17. It took her ten months to get better—but she did. You may recall how difficult it was for her to consent to treatment and how frustrating this was for her husband, Dick, and daughter, Patricia. Imagine how painfully long the ten-month course of treatment was for Irma and her family. Finally the treatment worked. Irma slowly improved and eventually marveled at her complete recovery; she was astounded to feel better than she had in many years. Irma told me how delighted she was to have the chance to get reacquainted with herself. She was eager to make up for lost time and quickly got busy living again.

The long ordeal that many of my patients, like Irma, go through before they get better is difficult for me, too. I have found that older adults and their family members have high expectations of what I can do for them. Some hope that I do actually have a "magic pill" that will make them better right away. Others have hung their hopes on antidepressant medication taking three to four weeks to work. Alas, all too often they are disappointed. Some will get better quickly, but for many it will take much longer. I hate giving them the bad news that treating their depression might take a lot longer than they thought.

But how long? Will it be weeks, months, or longer? I've found not being able to predict how long treatment will take, or whether it will even work at all, to be one of the most trying aspects of practicing geriatric psychiatry. It's hard not being able to relieve older patients' suffering right away.

So why does it sometimes take so long for patients such as Irma to get better? This is the so-called sixty-four-thousand-dollar question (the reference should be familiar to older readers). There is no simple answer, but it boils down to this: older adults, especially those in their late eighties and nineties, are more complicated, and their treatment is more challenging. In this chapter I am going to explain why treatment of older adults with depression can take so long. I have found that when my patients fully understand these reasons, they have an easier time sticking with treatment without losing hope. I hope this information will help you persevere until you, or your loved one, gets better.

GETTING THE DIAGNOSIS RIGHT

When you go to a doctor with a problem, you expect to get a diagnosis and leave with treatment. Older adults generally assume it ought to be that easy for depression, but often it is not so straightforward. Diagnosing depression takes time. If you are quickly given a prescription for depression, beware. You might not be getting the right treatment.

Doctors face three challenges in making a correct diagnosis. First, you might not actually have depression. A number of conditions masquerade as late-life depression. We covered these depression look-alikes in chapter 4. If what you have is one of these conditions, you might need an altogether different treatment. Whomever you see for professional help with depression might want you to see other specialists, such as neurologists or sleep specialists, before starting any treatment. This may take time.

Getting the wrong diagnosis wasn't a problem for Irma, but it was for Jerry. Jerry had very mild Alzheimer's disease, but he was doing a fine job managing on his own at home. Jerry's daughter Beth became concerned when she noticed a change in his behavior. Jerry lost interest in doing anything, stopped going out, and began spending almost all day in bed. This looked like depression to Beth. She took Jerry to his primary care physician and told him how depressed Jerry had become. Jerry's doctor prescribed an antidepressant.

The problem was, however, that Jerry didn't have depression. He had sleep apnea. This made him tired all the time. Because of his Alzheimer's, he simply concluded the right thing to do was stay in bed. Worse yet, the antidepressant medication the doctor prescribed made Jerry even more tired. Beth jumped to the wrong conclusion, understandably, about Jerry's having depression, and the doctor took her at face value. Given all the demands on primary care doctors these days, it's easy to see how this can happen. Don't let it happen to you. Don't jump to conclusions about what the problem is or agree to start treatment for depression before going through a thorough evaluation. There will be more on this in chapter 23.

The second challenge for doctors is correctly diagnosing the type of depression, when depression actually is the problem. Not all depression is the same. You may also remember the different diagnoses of depression we reviewed in chapter 4.

There is no one-size-fits-all treatment for depression, so getting the diagnosis right matters. Think of this as being akin to treating infections. Not all infections require an antibiotic. If you have a virus, not only is an antibiotic unnecessary; it may make you worse. If you have a bacterial infection, then your doctor needs to know what antibiotics it is sensitive to before prescribing for you. Similarly, not all types of depression require treatment with antidepressant medications. Some forms of depression do not require any treatment. Others respond very well to psychotherapy. And others definitely require medication. But in bipolar depression, antidepressants are usually a bad idea. They may help in the short run but make things worse in the long run. And in psychotic depression, an antipsychotic medication will be needed in addition to an antidepressant.

Sorting out these diagnostic questions may be possible during the first visit. But it might take two or more visits to arrive at the correct diagnosis of depression.

Why so long? The third challenge doctors face in diagnosing depression is the lack of tests for it. Other areas of medicine are not so handicapped. If you go to the emergency room with chest pain, the emergency doctor will order an electrocardiogram and blood work. Within minutes he or she will know whether you are having a heart attack (I hope you never have one). Without such tests, some patients actually having a heart attack might be sent home, where they could die, while others, with nothing more than heartburn, might be admitted to the coronary care unit.

A wrong diagnosis of depression can prove just as dire. We have already seen how Jerry was diagnosed incorrectly initially and received the wrong treatment. Getting the diagnosis of depression wrong can result in a suicidal person not getting the help needed. Or someone with bipolar depression might become manic and need to be hospitalized. And patients who could be treated successfully with psychotherapy might receive medication instead and develop serious side effects they might have been spared.

Unfortunately, to arrive at a correct diagnosis of depression, doctors must rely on patients' descriptions of their feelings, thoughts, and memories, and family members' observations of their loved one's behavior. It's not always easy to diagnose a problem from the subjective descriptions of others. Patients' descriptions of their current symptoms or their recollections of past histories can change from visit to visit. It's hard to remember everything in a doctor's office. People forget important details during the first visit, which they may not remember to mention until the second or third visit. It also takes a few visits for older adults to feel comfortable enough to disclose highly personal information.

I've found that some of my patients answer my questions differently on the second visit once they have gone home and had a chance to think about it. I may have asked them a question that jogged their memory. Much the same applies to family members. They sometimes describe their relatives' problems very differently in later visits.

An accurate description of past mental health problems is also important. This can make or break the current diagnosis of geriatric depression. Older adults often have trouble remembering details of problems and treatment that occurred decades in the past. Looking back, events blur together. Or people view them through rose-colored glasses. Some of my patients know that they took medications for depression in the past but cannot remember the names of the drugs. Others recall having been hospitalized for a "nervous breakdown" but can't be more descriptive than that. Depression and poor memory make it even harder to recall the past accurately.

Think about it. Do you remember how you felt one year ago? How about just last week? Can you describe it to yourself, in words that would give others a clear picture? You don't have to practice medicine for very long to realize how hard it is for even highly motivated, diligent patients and family members to get the story right the first time. Often it is necessary to obtain prior medical records or to speak to family members who are not immediately available. This all takes time.

Most patients are better off in the long run when their doctors take the time needed to get the diagnosis right. This is far better than rushing into treatment only to discover later that it's the wrong treatment. This wastes more time and exposes patients to unnecessary risks.

DOUBTS AND HESITATION

Once the doctor feels confident about the diagnosis of depression and recommends a course of treatment, getting started may still take some time, as it did with Irma. I won't go through it all again. You may wish to reread chapter 17 to refresh your memory of Irma, her many doubts about antidepressant medications, and how she tenaciously dragged her heels about taking one. Eventually she did start medication, but her hesitation delayed the start of treatment for many weeks.

Many older adults are reluctant to accept any form of psychiatric treatment, and it takes time to help them resolve their doubts. Barring life-threatening emergencies, there's no way around this. Older adults cannot be rushed. Medical treatment of any kind rarely succeeds when patients don't accept that it is in their interest to have it. It either doesn't work or actually backfires.

INCREASED SENSITIVITY TO MEDICATION

Irma finally started taking her medication. We crossed our fingers and hoped that her treatment would go smoothly. Alas, it was not to be. Within one week Irma fainted. She was taken to the hospital emergency room and admitted overnight for observation. Fortunately everything was okay. A slew of tests turned up nothing. Because no other cause for the fainting spell could be found, I had to assume the new medication was the culprit, so I stopped it.

As we age, our bodies become more sensitive to medications, both their helpful actions and their side effects. This means that older adults usually require less medication than do younger people. Medical textbooks say that older adults require one-half to one-third the standard adult dose for most medications. Geriatric psychiatrists, including me, tend to be more cautious. We usually start our patients with one-tenth to one-fifth of the standard dose. I had started Irma on a very small dose, a smidgen really. Irma's setback illustrates how sensitive older patients can be to even very tiny doses of medication.

Side effects that might be little more than a nuisance to younger people can be serious for older adults. Irma could have been hurt when she fainted. I think you can see how older adults' greater sensitivity to medications leads to more false starts in their treatment. We try to prevent such delays and complications by prescribing very low doses to begin with. Obviously, this strategy does not always work.

Thankfully, despite Irma's initial reservations about taking medication, she was willing to try another one, even after being hospitalized with an apparent side effect. Irma was allergic to the next medication I prescribed. It gave her a red, itchy rash, and I had to stop that medicine, too.

Allergies and side effects are different kettles of fish. Side effects are caused by the known actions of medications. They are predictable. We know that a certain percentage of patients, hopefully a very small one, will develop some side effects of a medication. In many cases, we also know that the higher the dose, the more people will get side effects and the more severe they will be. This is one important reason we take extra time to find the lowest dose that does the job.

In contrast, allergies are not related to how drugs work. Instead, they come from individuals' natural immune defenses. Allergies are not predictable, which means they are always a surprise, and nothing can be done to prevent them.

Things went more smoothly with the third medication. To use a baseball metaphor, not wanting to strike out, I protected the plate. I gave Irma one-tenth of the dose I thought she would need to get better.

Not until two weeks later, once I was sure the medication agreed with her, did I raise the dose by another tenth.

Why was there so much time between dose adjustments? Medications accumulate more slowly in older adults. After any dose increase, the amount of medication in the body gradually accumulates until a new plateau is reached. This may take a week or two—even longer with some medications. It's not until this plateau is reached that we truly know whether or not there are side effects. It is best to wait at least this long before considering further dose increases.

INTERACTIONS

My patients often ask me whether a medication I've recommended to them is going to interact with their other medications. They are right to be concerned. Older adults take more medications than do younger people. The more medications you take, the higher the likelihood of a drug interaction happening. It is not always possible to completely avoid drug interactions. Beginning with very small amounts of medication and raising the dose slowly is the best way to ensure that if there is a drug interaction it will be spotted before any serious problem occurs.

DELAYED RESPONSE

People suffering from depression want and need quick relief, but antidepressant medications take time to work. Because of this, they are not great medications, but they are what we have.

Older adults respond nearly as well to treatment of depression as do younger patients, but it usually takes much longer. The time it takes for antidepressant medications to work is called the response latency. Old age makes this waiting period longer. My patients have heard that antidepressant medications take three to four weeks to "kick in." It would be nice if it were only that bad. The response delay for older patients can be as long as twelve weeks. As important as it is to be patient for treatment to work, twelve weeks is much too long to wait to see whether an antidepressant medication is going to work or not.

In trying to help my patients, I, like most geriatric psychiatrists, try to strike a balance between speed and safety. To avoid prescribing a higher dose than is necessary, I usually try to give a medication enough time to see whether it is going to work before raising the dose. Waiting about one month is about the right compromise. If patients have improved significantly by then, waiting longer for further improvement is often a good idea. Two or three months later they may be completely better. They won't need more medication. But if there has been little or no improvement by a month, then raising the dose is reasonable. Waiting that month allows the doctor and the patient to feel fairly confident that raising the dose is the right thing to do.

"START LOW, GO SLOW"

To compensate for the greater sensitivity to medication, longer response latency, and higher chance of drug interactions, geriatric psychiatrists use an approach known as "start low, go slow" in prescribing medications, including antidepressants. We begin treatment with a very low dose of medication (start low). Think of it as putting a toe in the water rather than diving in. If no improvement occurs after a few weeks, we raise the dose by a similarly small amount, as I described before. This process is patiently repeated (go slow) until the patient gets better, develops side effects, or "maxes out" on the medication. While many older adults respond to very low doses of medication, some turn out to need doses as high as do younger people. In this case, "start low, go slow" turns into "start low, go slow, go all the way."

"Start low, go slow" is a pretty good way of finding the lowest amount of medication that works while avoiding the temptation to rush into higher doses than necessary. As you can imagine, this can be a lengthy process. It can feel tedious. It requires patience, which can be tough. But it's tried and true.

TRIAL-AND-ERROR NATURE OF TREATMENT

Here's another built-in problem that can drag out treatment. Not all patients respond to all medications. Individuals respond to some medications but not others. This applies to many different types of medications, not only antidepressants.

For example, let's consider treatment of high cholesterol. There are five or six available cholesterol-lowering medications, known as statins. All work about the same but not for everyone. Lipitor might do a great job lowering your cholesterol but not mine. I might get good results with Crestor, but you might not. There's no way to know in advance.

The same is true of antidepressant medications. They are all equally effective, on average, but we do not know how well any single medication will work for any individual. A culture and sensitivity test can tell which antibiotics will kill a bacterial infection, but medical science has not yet provided us with a similar tool for depression. We have no surefire method to predict which antidepressant medication will be best for an individual. Doctors use their experience, judgment, and knowledge of medications to choose antidepressants they think will have the best chance of helping their patients. But in the end, there is still some trial and error to it.

To return to a metaphor I used before, look at it this way. Imagine you are standing in front of a locked door that you need to open. Actually this is a pretty good analogy, since depression really locks its victims in. Now further imagine that you have a key ring with thirty keys on it, but you have no idea which one unlocks the door. There is no master key. The best you can do is to try them one at a time until you come upon the one that unlocks the door. Maybe you can inspect the lock and narrow the possibilities down to ten keys, based on their shape. Treatment of depression is very much akin to this. Doctors' key rings have twenty or more antidepressant medications on them. The good news is that more than one antidepressant may open the depression lock—several might. But we have no way to know in advance which key or keys will unlock the door. The first few you try might not unlock the depression.

Patients may have to try two, three, four, or more antidepressants before arriving at one that works, each time following the start low, go slow process. Each false start can delay treatment by several weeks, with no guarantee of success at the end. But with perseverance treatment succeeds more often than not.

So far we have looked at aspects of treating depression that are out of your control. To recap, the doctor's job is to get you better. He or she must be cautious, above all, but also systematic, thorough, and relent-less. Your job is to get better. To accomplish this you need to under-stand the game plan, that is, how treatment works and what to expect, and be as patient as you can to deal with the delays that occur.

Knowing what to expect helps. Travelers from New York to New Zealand can expect a long trip, nearly twenty-four hours. Knowing it will take this long helps them prepare so that it isn't more unpleasant than need be. They also know they will get to their destination. A three-hour layover you anticipate is less upsetting than a three-hour delay you didn't. Treatment of geriatric depression can be a long-distance jour-ney. Understanding the types of layovers and delays that occur along the way makes you a better passenger.

If you have begun taking a new medication and feel only a glimmer of improvement after one or two weeks, do not be discouraged. Resist the temptation to abandon the medication as ineffective. Instead, see the glimmer, even if it is only a 10 percent improvement, as a sign the medication is working, and report this to your doctor as objectively as you can. It may be easier for family members to notice small improve-ments and objectively report them to your doctor, so they have an important role in your treatment.

We now turn to delays related to interruptions of treatment—delays you can do something about.

REGULAR FOLLOW-UP APPOINTMENTS

Regular appointments are essential for treatment of depression to suc-ceed. Once treatment starts, it is a good idea to have a follow-up visit fairly soon to keep things moving ahead smoothly. If you have started taking an antidepressant medication, don't let too much time elapse before seeing your doctor again, as did Larry.

Larry was a seventy-eight-year-old retired chemist who had been widowed five years. He'd been in fairly good health and had been well until he developed depression. Larry went to see his primary care doc-tor, who prescribed 25 mg of the antidepressant medication sertraline, the generic name for Zoloft. Larry took the medication faithfully but did not get better. Larry's primary care doctor did not make a follow-up appointment, assuming Larry would return if he didn't respond. Larry didn't return. Because he was old, Larry didn't expect to get better and so didn't know why he should bother.

Ten months later, Larry's daughter, Arlene, brought Larry to see me. I evaluated Larry and came to a number of conclusions. Larry had a type of depression called major depressive disorder. His primary care physician had chosen a good medication and had started a low dose. So far, so good. But he didn't go slow; in fact, he didn't go at all. There was no follow-up, and ten months later Larry was still taking the same low starting dose and was no better. I simply increased the dose to 50 mg. Within one week, Larry responded. One month later, at the appointment I made for him, he felt like "a new man." Arlene thought I was a genius, but she deserved the real credit for taking action and getting treatment rolling again.

Larry's case illustrates another reason I consider geriatric depression to be a family illness. Family members have an important role in treatment and often make the difference in its success. Had Larry had another appointment a few weeks after his first visit to his primary care physician, he might have been back to normal in about one month instead of eleven. As we will now see, family members can have an important role in keeping other barriers from delaying treatment. If you are having or considering treatment for depression, be mindful of barriers that may delay your progress, and let family members, or others you trust, help you circumvent them.

UNEXPECTED ILLNESS

Back to Irma. She seemed cursed. Six weeks into treatment with the third medication we tried she got pneumonia. She was hospitalized for four days and then went to rehab for two weeks. Because of a potential interaction with the antibiotics she needed, her antidepressant was stopped. She missed her scheduled appointment with me. By the time she was well enough to come to my office, six weeks had gone by and she was still off her antidepressant. We were able to get back on track, but this added up to a two-month setback.

Older adults are more prone to get sick than are younger people. Health problems, big and small, crop up. Respiratory infections, diarrheal illness, urinary tract infections, injuries from falls, and flare-ups of emphysema, congestive heart failure, or diabetes can waylay older adults and interrupt treatment of their depression.

If you are hospitalized for an illness, make sure the hospital doctor knows you have started a medication for depression and what the dose is. Do not assume the list the hospital has is up to date. If the hospital doctor stopped your antidepressant, make sure your regular doctor knows the medical reasons. Once you return home, do not let too much time go by before getting a new appointment to resume treatment for your depression.

COGNITIVE IMPAIRMENT

Lapses in memory, attention, and concentration are frequent symptoms of late-life depression. Family members often tell me they've noticed that their loved one seems to be not thinking straight. They get concerned about bad decisions based on sketchy judgment.

Impairment of cognitive abilities and thinking can be part of late-life depression, and it can lead to avoidable glitches in treatment. These include forgetting to keep appointments, forgetting to take medications, or getting the directions for taking medications wrong. Such problems can derail treatment pretty quickly. They derailed Irma.

When I prescribed the third medication for Irma, Patricia asked me to send the prescription to a pharmacy near her office to make it easier for her to pick up her mother's prescriptions. The family forgot to tell the original pharmacy that the first medication had been stopped. One month later, that pharmacy automatically refilled Irma's old prescription and called Irma to tell her it was ready. In the fog of depression, she assumed she was supposed to take it, which she did, along with the new medication. The two drugs interacted to cause symptoms that didn't make sense to me. It was almost ten days before Irma's husband realized what had happened, but in the meantime I had stopped Irma's new antidepressant. We quickly got things back on track, but this set her back another two weeks.

Don't let this happen to you or someone you love. Use a buddy system. Don't be too proud to rely on a helper. Older adults sometimes feel reluctant to accept this type of help. Depression makes many patients feel helpless. Some cope with the insecurity they feel by turning down needed assistance. I'm sure you know the adage "two heads are better than one." It's really apt here. Think of your helper as a copilot or wingman. If there is no one in the family who can serve this function, consider hiring a geriatric case manager until you get better.

BAD WEATHER

Snow, ice, torrential rain, heavy smog, and heat waves can all be hazardous to frail older adults. When bad weather poses a safety risk, staying indoors is advisable; and canceling appointments, prudent. Missing an appointment for treating depression is a setback, but a broken hip from falling on the ice or a hospitalization for heat stroke are much bigger setbacks. This is a time to cut your losses and stay safe. If you are not sure what to do, rely on your copilot's judgment.

LOGISTICS

About one-third of my patients drive themselves to their appointments. The rest no longer drive at all or, because of depression, do not feel confident behind the wheel.

Irma had not driven in over a year. Dick handled all the local driving, but the trip to my office took forty minutes, and it involved interstate highways, too much for him to handle. Patricia had to take off work to bring her mom to see me. The best-case scenario meant being away from her job for three hours. After the sixth appointment in five months, Patricia's boss became impatient with this, and Patricia was afraid of being fired. She canceled Irma's next appointment and then told me she'd be unable to come more frequently than every two months. Fortunately, a neighbor was able to help out, and Irma's treatment stayed on track.

Transportation difficulties pose another barrier to the progress of treatment for depression. Having to depend on others for rides is not easy. It compounds helpless feelings. Older adults often feel guilty about asking their busy children for rides. They do not want to inconvenience them. There's no easy way around this problem. Drivers, no matter how well meaning and responsible, are sometimes not completely reliable. Older spouses themselves get sick. They may not be well enough to drive. They may need to see their own doctors, and their problems may be more urgent. Children face competing demands. They may have parenting responsibilities that take priority or jobs they cannot easily leave. It's not uncommon for my patients to cancel appointments at the last minute because a son or daughter had to take an unexpected business trip.

The best-laid plans of mice and men . . . Just as older adults will miss a certain number of appointments due to hazardous weather, they will also miss visits due to breakdowns of transportation plans. This is par for the course. There may not be much to be done about this other than hope it happens no more than once in the course of treatment. If you think this may be a bigger problem, one thing you can do is line up a backup driver. If your doctor's office is nearby, your town may have a senior van you can use.

CONCLUSION

Few patients face as many complications as did Irma. Most patients' cases resemble Agnes's more, although few patients complete treatment without running into at least one delay. Looking back, it's amazing that it did not take longer than ten months for Irma to get better.

There are other things you can do to avoid delays in your treatment or that of your loved one. Try not to ask your doctor for tranquilizers or sleeping pills for quick relief while you wait for your antidepressant to start working. Seeking quick relief for these symptoms invites the complications we try to avoid with start low, go slow. Try to be patient. Once your antidepressant starts working, you'll sleep better and feel less anxious. Keep regular appointments. Make sure that visits with your doctor occur frequently enough to make progress. Don't do what Larry did. If you are not getting better, and you have not seen your doctor for some time, get an appointment as soon as possible. Take care of yourself. Eat well. Exercise, if you are physically well enough. And make sure to take care of your other health problems, such as diabetes.

I hope your response to treatment is closer to Agnes's than to Irma's. But even if it is not, keep in mind that Irma did get better. If you persevere with treatment, you will too. The moral of Aesop's fable "The

Tortoise and the Hare," "slow and steady wins the race," applies well in treatment of older adults with depression. It has been two years, and Irma has remained well. Treatment worked, and she got her life back, and you can too. If you stick with the treatment, the odds are in your favor.

22

THE SHOCKING FACTS ABOUT
SHOCK TREATMENT

I don't like introducing the topic with my patients, and I thought twice about including it here. But those few patients who need to hear about it really do, and maybe you do as well. I'm talking about electroconvulsive therapy, ECT for short.

When I introduce this subject to patients and members of their families, they usually give me quizzical looks. When I clarify that I am referring to "shock treatment," the expressions turn to surprise and horror: surprise, because most people are shocked (pun intended) to learn that shock treatment is still used in the twenty-first century; and horror as they realize I am suggesting it as a possible treatment for them. It's never an easy discussion. But it's a crucial one. For older adults stuck in severe, debilitating depression, from which there seems no escape, shock treatment may be their last, best hope to get their lives back. That is why we still use it and why you should know about it.

"IT'S NOT YOUR FATHER'S OLDSMOBILE"

Remember my very reluctant patient Irma from chapters 17 and 21? Convincing her to agree to take antidepressant medications was extremely challenging. Ring a bell? Well, that was nothing compared to the challenge of convincing older adults to have shock treatment. Most often they reject it immediately. Getting them just to listen, much less keep an open mind, can be very tough. Most are terrified of it. And I understand why. But here's the thing. Once they have had their first treatment, they tell me it was a "piece of cake" or "no big deal." Some wonder why they had been so scared.

Older adults have been around long enough to recall decades-old horror stories of family members or friends who had shock treatment in the days of the old asylums. The 1975 film *One Flew Over the Cuckoo's Nest* depicts how ECT was administered back then. Such gruesome images of shock treatment have been etched indelibly in the minds of the public and are what patients fear when ECT is recommended to them.

Shock treatment remains one of, if not the most, stigmatized treatment in all of medicine—undeservedly so. It evokes visceral fear and loathing. And, yet, after patients have their first treatment, they often remark that it was not as bad as they had imagined. This chapter will help you understand why shock treatment is used for older people, how the treatment is done, what is known about its benefits, and the risks.

WHO RECEIVES ECT?

Very few patients receive ECT any longer. Because ECT works quickly and reliably, it provides the speedier response needed in life-threatening depression. Some depressed patients are so determined to die that it may be difficult to prevent them from committing suicide or starving themselves to death. It may not be safe to wait for medications to work in such situations.

ECT is also used to treat moderately to severely depressed patients who are not responding to other treatments. Think of it as a last resort in such cases. And ECT is used very rarely to prevent severely ill patients in an agitated frenzy from inadvertently hurting themselves.

WHY ECT IS STILL USED

Electroconvulsive therapy has been around since 1938. It was discovered by accident when doctors noticed that patients with both depression and epilepsy temporarily got better after epileptic convulsions.

Doctors learned that they could bring about the same improvement by inducing convulsions artificially, using various medical means. For the first time, something could be done for patients with untreatable, serious depression.

Eighty years later we still use ECT because this strange treatment works better than any other treatment we have for severe depression. And it works faster. ECT is 90 percent effective for older people with severe depression, a pretty impressive success rate. However, if many attempts with different combinations of medications have failed, ECT's effectiveness may drop to 50 to 60 percent.[1] All in all, older patients treated with ECT are twice as likely to experience complete relief of symptoms and full recovery of function as those who receive other treatments.

WHAT IS ECT AND HOW IS IT DONE?

As the name implies, ECT involves using electricity to cause a medically controlled convulsion for therapeutic benefit. ECT is usually done in a specialized area of a hospital set up for the purpose. This may be a recovery room or other area near the operating suite. The team of professionals involved in the treatment typically includes the ECT psychiatrist, an anesthesiologist or nurse anesthetist, and a recovery nurse. The ECT psychiatrist is in charge of the treatment itself. The anesthesia professional induces sleep and ensures medical safety throughout. The recovery nurse assists patients through the treatment until they are ready to leave.

Except for the insertion of an intravenous line, ECT is completely painless. Patients are fully asleep for the entire treatment, which takes only a few minutes. After being put to sleep with a very short-acting anesthetic, a muscle relaxant is given to prevent a physical convulsion. A physical convulsion is not necessary for ECT to work as long as an electrical seizure in the brain occurs. Other medications are given to prevent the heart from slowing down too much. Patients with certain kinds of heart conditions may also receive medications to prevent the heart from speeding up. Next, an electrical shock sufficient to induce a seizure is applied to the scalp. The duration of the electrical shock is from less than a full second to a few seconds at most. This induces an electrical seizure in the brain. The seizure lasts about forty-five seconds on average. During this time, heart rate, blood pressure, breathing, and seizure activity are monitored. If the seizure lasts more than three minutes, medications are given to bring it to a halt. After a few minutes, patients wake up. Usually they remain groggy for a few more minutes and are temporarily disoriented and confused. This clears up rapidly.

ECT is usually given two to three times per week. Patients may be admitted to the hospital, but these days more ECT is done as an outpatient treatment. A course of ECT typically includes seven to eight treatments. Sometimes fewer are enough, but more may be needed as well. It is the job of the ECT psychiatrist to monitor patients' progress, ensure that the treatments are well tolerated, and decide when enough treatments have been given.

A course of ECT is often stopped once the depression gets better. In some cases, ECT is tapered off rather than stopped abruptly. Patients may receive a few weekly treatments after which the treatments are tapered to biweekly and then monthly, until they are stopped entirely.

If depression comes back fairly soon, and ECT must be resumed, the treating psychiatrist may recommend maintenance treatments. Maintenance ECT is almost always done as an outpatient. Treatments are administered as often as needed to keep symptoms from returning. Commonly this is once a month.[2]

ECT can be either unilateral or bilateral. Unilateral means that the shock is applied to only one side of the head, usually the right side in right-handed people. Bilateral treatment is applied to both sides of the head. Bilateral treatment is usually more effective. Unilateral treatment is less likely to cause confusion, delirium, or memory impairment. Most often doctors begin a course of ECT with unilateral treatment. They will switch to bilateral treatment if there is no sign of improvement.

HOW DOES ECT WORK?

How ECT works was a mystery for decades. Researchers recently discovered, using modern, high-tech brain-scanning tools, that ECT restores normal function in brain circuits affected in depression. Exactly how ECT does this remains unknown. When medicine works, it has the same effect. Remarkably, unlike medication, which does not work quite as well for older people as for younger people, ECT works better for the elderly.

IS ECT SAFE?

ECT is riskier for older patients than younger patients, but this is true of the vast majority of medical treatment. And ECT is one of the safest medical treatments done under anesthesia. Research has shown that ECT is safe for patients over age eighty-five.[3] And for many older patients, ECT may be safer than taking medications for depression.[4] Older patients may get better results with ECT and with fewer side effects than medication.

Many people worry that ECT causes brain damage or permanent memory impairment, but this is not the case. Medical researchers have been conducting extensive studies for decades to look for evidence of these adverse effects without being able to find any proof that either occurs. As you can imagine, because ECT is controversial, such concerns have prompted much research. In fact, ECT is one of the most thoroughly researched treatments in all of modern medicine.

What about memory impairment? Most patients have some cognitive side effects. These are usually tolerable and do not interfere with continuing treatment. The confusion that occurs after each treatment is the most common side effect. Patients wake up from the anesthesia feeling disoriented and confused. It takes five minutes to an hour for this to clear up. Sometimes the confusion is severe enough that further treatment has to be delayed for a time. One study of patients over eighty-five found that their cognitive abilities, on average, improved after successful treatment with ECT.[5]

Anterograde amnesia is one form of memory disturbance that ECT commonly causes. This refers to the ability to form new memories, and patients often find it disturbing. Anterograde amnesia typically goes away after one to three weeks. Retrograde amnesia can also occur. This involves loss of memory for things that happened before the treatment. The period of time affected can be one to three months. Some memories will return, but some may not. Sometimes it is difficult to separate memory impairment caused by ECT from the memory impairment caused by depression. Patients with cognitive impairment due to depression actually show an improvement in memory and cognitive abilities after successful treatment with ECT.

Some older adults are under the misunderstanding that ECT works by causing a stroke. This occurs in regions where older people refer to a stroke as "a shock." Because they know ECT as "shock treatment," they equate the two. This connection leads to unnecessary confusion and alarm. Fortunately, ECT has nothing to do with having a stroke. In fact, older people with depression have an increased risk of having a stroke, and successful treatment of depression lowers this risk. So ECT may lessen the chance of having a stroke.

ECT is not safe for everyone. Anyone who has recently had a heart attack cannot have ECT. People with serious abnormalities of their heart rhythm may not be able to have it. Individuals with congestive heart failure cannot have ECT until the congestive heart failure is under control. And people with brain diseases associated with increased pressure in and around the brain cannot have ECT. ECT can be given to people with Alzheimer's disease and related disorders, and people who have had a stroke in the past can have it.

CONCLUSION

In its heyday, ECT was extensively used. The discovery of antidepressant medications offered an effective, more acceptable alternative for most patients with depression, and ECT use became infrequent. These days ECT is used to treat older adults with depression only after exhaustive treatment with medication has failed. Doctors consider turning to ECT sooner when a fast response is needed to help people who are extremely suicidal, dangerously agitated, or deteriorating physically from depression. For some suffering older adults, ECT is their last hope to get better. For others, it can be lifesaving.

23

GETTING THE TREATMENT YOU NEED

Being an Educated Consumer

Thank God we found you!" "Do you have any idea what we went through before someone suggested we come here?" "Why didn't anyone tell us that there are specialists called geriatric psychiatrists?" These are typical of the sentiments my patients or their family members express when they meet me. Their relief is palpable. Many wash up on my shores having been lost at sea in the healthcare system, adrift with depression and unable to find a helpful port.

Okay, so I just got a little corny and melodramatic. But if you have been struggling to get help for depression, maybe you understand why. Sadly, the vast majority of older adults with depression receive either no treatment or ineffective treatment.[1] Why? Because geriatric mental health specialists are very, very scarce. Most older adults with depression have no access to one. And the rest of the healthcare system doesn't have a clue about the special needs of older patients with mental health problems. Harsh words? You bet! But it's not just my opinion. The Institute of Medicine thinks so, too, and it is the nation's healthcare brain trust.[2]

I don't mean to scare you away, having spent the better part of a whole book trying to convince you to have treatment for depression. And we don't have a lousy healthcare system. But two of its weaknesses happen to be geriatrics and mental health, a double whammy for older adults, and this is why the treatment they receive for depression often falls short. You still can get good treatment, but you have to know what to look for. You must become an educated consumer. This chapter will give you a head start.

IT'S NOT CALLED PRIMARY CARE FOR NOTHING

The vast majority of older adults who receive treatment for depression get it from their primary care physician. In general, older adults are more comfortable seeing their primary care doctors than mental health specialists. So if you have depression and want to get professional help, where should you start? It depends on what resources for help are available in your area. If a geriatric psychiatrist has hung a shingle in your neighborhood, you could start there. Or you might decide to see a psychologist or another type of psychotherapist, if you think psycho-therapy would be your best bet. Either choice would be okay, but I'd prefer that you see your primary care physician first. Why?

First, unless you are extremely fortunate, there isn't a geriatric psychiatrist in your neighborhood, or anywhere remotely close. These subspecialists ought to be on the endangered species list; they are in critically short supply.

Second, it's almost always a mistake to start any psychiatric treat-ment without first getting a complete physical checkup. An underactive thyroid, or other medical condition, might be causing your depression. Talking to a psychotherapist might seem like the right thing to do, but correcting the thyroid problem, or other underlying medical cause, is a higher priority. It may relieve your depression. And until this is done, psychotherapy may not be of much help.

Your primary care physician already knows you and your medical history. He or she can easily test you for the common medical causes of depression. If you need antidepressant medication, your primary care physician can prescribe it for you. Most primary care doctors prescribe antidepressants, and they are usually fairly cautious, a good thing. Sometimes they are too cautious. More on this later. If your depression is on the milder side, and your health is not too complicated, your primary care doctor may be all you need to get better. So let's look at what should and should not happen in primary care treatment of geriat-ric depression.

First, it is very important that the doctor spends time taking a careful history of your depression. In chapter 4, we covered how complicated and confusing diagnosis of late-life depression can be. It takes time to decide that an older adult has depression and that it's the type that can benefit from medication. Some primary care doctors do not take the time needed to make the correct diagnosis.[3] They react to symptoms without getting to the bottom of them. This is asking for trouble. You might receive the wrong treatment for the wrong diagnosis. So if you receive a prescription for an antidepressant minutes after mentioning that you feel depressed, beware.

READY, FIRE, AIM

Lenore came to me for a second opinion. Her primary care doctor had prescribed an antidepressant during a routine office visit, but she didn't think she needed it and didn't want to take it. She was right. Lenore's husband died two years earlier, but she had mourned successfully and was doing fine.

During her annual checkup, Lenore's doctor asked what was going on in her life. When she mentioned that her children had convinced her to sell the house and move to a condominium, she cried briefly. The doctor was warm and sympathetic but didn't ask any further questions about her emotional state. So Lenore was surprised when, at the end of her appointment, the doctor wrote her a prescription for an antidepressant and told her he wanted her to take it.

Lenore left feeling bewildered. She hadn't thought she had depression. "But I'm no doctor," she explained to me. You also have to wonder about her primary care doctor. In fact Lenore didn't have depression. What she did have was the prior loss of her husband; an unsettling, stressful move in the near future; and a momentary emotional outburst. By themselves, these do not add up to depression and are not reasons to take medication, or necessarily to have any treatment.

In another case, a patient's daughter called the primary care doctor concerned that her mother was depressed. She wondered whether there was something her mother could take for it. Without further ado, the doctor phoned in a prescription for an antidepressant to the pharmacy. Shame on the daughter; shame on the doctor. This patient needed treatment but not for depression—for kidney failure. Patients are better off with no treatment than this type of treatment. Never accept treatment prescribed solely on the basis of a symptom you (or a member of your family) report, especially over the phone or by e-mail. This goes as well for psychotherapy, which should not be recommended until your doctor has checked you over to make sure you have depression and it is not caused by one of the many other conditions that masquerade as depression.

Frances was a retired college English professor who was depressed. She had divorced three husbands but never fell out of love with books, the true love of her life. In old age, her body let her down. Macular degeneration left her legally blind and unable to read, and crippling arthritis forced her to live with her daughter. Frances became very depressed. Her primary care physician took a history and diagnosed major depressive disorder. He concluded that Frances's losses were more than she could bear, and he referred her to a psychotherapist. Unfortunately, eight sessions of talk therapy helped not one bit, so Frances came to me for a second opinion.

After meeting Frances, I agreed she had depression. But she was also taking two blood pressure medications that can cause depression. And no blood work had been done. I ordered the needed tests and discovered she had vitamin B_{12} deficiency and hypothyroidism. Once these problems were corrected and she was taken off the blood pressure medications, she felt like herself again. She had the same tough-to-swallow losses but no longer had depression.

DOS AND DON'TS TO WATCH FOR

Have I puzzled you? After touting primary care physicians as your first stop for treatment, I just gave you three examples of errors they might make. Many primary care physicians do a good job. If yours does, great; you're all set. But you need to know how to tell when he or she isn't up to snuff, at least for your depression. Let's go over what you should look for.

We will start with the examination. What goes into a good one? In addition to a head-to-toe physical examination, which should include checks of reflexes, strength, balance, and walking, the doctor ought to ask you a few questions to test your memory and other cognitive abilities. He or she should review all your medications, including over-the-counter products and herbal and nutritional supplements (remember to tell your doctor about these), to determine whether any could be a factor in your depression. And he or she should order blood tests, including routine blood counts and chemistries, thyroid tests, and levels of vitamins B_{12}, D, and folic acid.

Now, let's say you have depression and need an antidepressant and your doctor has given you a prescription for one. Problem solved? Hardly. The majority of older adults treated for depression in primary care fail to respond to the first medication prescribed.[4] If this happens to you, don't give up! Better results are possible, but you must pursue it.

Too often in American medicine this does not happen. Patients get a prescription and are told to return if they don't get better. This doesn't work. Remember Larry from chapter 21? He was given a low dose of Zoloft but had no follow-up, and ten months later he was still depressed. Frequent, regular appointments are needed to monitor your progress to make sure that treatment is working and on track. If you are not getting better, the treatment should be adjusted every one to four weeks.

Your doctor should be vigilant about side effects, and this requires seeing you often. Doing so, he or she might be able to identify side effects early, possibly before you are aware you have them, and take steps to keep them from becoming trouble for you.

Frequent appointments are also important so your doctor can answer all your questions. Many questions come up in the course of treating depression. Even with appointments as often as weekly, there are always new questions. They are all important and they all need to be answered. Getting timely answers goes a long way toward putting older adults' minds at ease. But when questions fester too long, they can snowball into the types of worries and doubts my patient Irma had. It's important that you understand your treatment and feel comfortable with it. A sign of good treatment is that your doctor takes the time for this.

So if rule number one was "don't accept treatment without a proper evaluation," rule number two is "don't accept treatment without scheduling another appointment fairly soon." If your doctor does not feel it is needed, ask to make it anyway, for your peace of mind.

Once you feel well, you still need to keep regular appointments. Just because things seem back to normal doesn't mean complications can't still occur. They can and they do, all the time, in all kinds of unexpected ways. By seeing you regularly your doctor can catch these while the fuse is still burning and prevent the explosion from blowing up in your face.

DON'T WAIT FOR THE COWS TO COME HOME

Waiting ten months before raising the dose of your antidepressant is obviously way too long. So how long should you wait before asking your doctor about a dose increase? If you are taking an adequate dose of antidepressant, then it takes twelve weeks to be sure it's not going to work.

Twelve weeks is a long time to wait when you don't feel well. And how do you know whether the dose is adequate? An adequate dose is the amount of medication that will make many older adults better. I know, that's vague. Depending on whom you ask, you might get different answers. You can ask your doctor whether the dose you began is a low, starting dose or a standard, therapeutic dose. For example, 25 mg of sertraline is a starting dose. Some older adults will respond to it. Most will need 50 mg, the standard therapeutic dose.

What's important is that if you are not responding, regardless of the dose, you need to ask your doctor about a dose increase or another change of treatment. Many psychiatrists will start with a low dose, but if there is no sign of improvement in two weeks, they will nudge the dose up. Others may prefer to wait a full month. If you are not at least 40 percent better after a month, you should expect some change in treatment.[5]

MORE RULES OF THUMB

A third useful rule of thumb is, "If you think you have bipolar disorder (see chapter 4), be wary of taking antidepressants for depression." True, antidepressants relieve depression in those with bipolar disorder. But in doing this, they can also trigger a switch into mania. It is preferable for patients with bipolar depression to be treated for this with a group of medications called mood stabilizers. Antidepressant medications can be added if the mood stabilizer has not helped the depression. Having a mood stabilizer in place may prevent mania from occurring.

Rule of thumb number four is "try to avoid taking benzodiazepines" (or "benzos"). Back a few chapters, when we covered medications, we began discussing the problems with these tranquilizers, which include the familiar brand names Xanax, Ativan, Klonopin, and Valium. Patients with depression often have severe anxiety. They prefer benzos because they provide relief within minutes. I find that patients already on benzos do not want to take antidepressants because they don't feel any immediate effect from them. Many of them tell me that their benzo is "the only pill that helps me." It's hard to convince them otherwise, and benzos do not treat depression.

Here's the problem with benzos. In the long run, you still have depression plus a new problem: you are addicted to your benzo. When I point out this risk, my patients ask, "Why does addiction matter at my age?" Good question. No, I'm not worried you'll try to score drugs on a downtown street corner or "knock over" a liquor store to support your habit. I am worried that using benzos increases the rate of falls and hip fractures, and causes or worsens cognitive impairment. These are high prices to pay for a medication that does not treat your depression and will be difficult or impossible for you to stop taking. This is trouble you can avoid.

The last rule of thumb is "don't sell yourself short." Set your goal of treatment to be back to normal. Too many older adults don't expect to get better because they think depression is just part of aging and the elderly don't respond well to treatment. Others settle for halfway improvement. While some improvement is better than none, and is often the best that can be done, don't compromise too soon. If your primary care physician tells you there's nothing more he or she can do, consider seeing a specialist if you can.

How might seeing a specialist help? Maybe your diagnosis is wrong. You might have bipolar depression or psychotic depression, or one of the masqueraders. Maybe you need a higher dose of medication than your primary care physician is comfortable prescribing. Or you might need a specialized combination of medication to break the logjam. Adding psychotherapy to your medication might do the trick, or possibly introducing an integrative therapy, such as fish oil, folate, or exercise, if you haven't done so already.

GETTING NOWHERE? WHERE DO YOU LOOK NEXT?

Some primary care doctors do not treat depression at all, and yours might tell you right off the bat to see a psychiatrist. Most do treat depression, and as I said earlier, this may be all you need. But what if it's not? When should your primary care doctor refer you to a specialist? If you have taken two different antidepressants, each for twelve weeks at adequate dose, and you are not better, referral is a good idea. So where do you go next? Lets look at the various healthcare professionals who are involved in treating geriatric depression so you can get a better idea of what they can and cannot do to help. Which one you see may depend on availability in your area.

Geriatric Psychiatrists

Call me biased, but geriatric psychiatrists are the gold standard. Psychiatrists are medical doctors, so they understand how to treat patients with physical, mental, and emotional problems. Geriatric psychiatrists have additional training in the diagnosis and treatment of older adults. They understand the interaction of depression and other health problems; are familiar with drugs older people take for their physical illnesses and the mental and emotional side effects they cause; can prescribe antidepressants and other medications; and perform psychotherapy. They are the most highly qualified specialists to treat older adults with depression.

Unfortunately, geriatric psychiatrists are few and far between, and you may not have access to one. But if you beat the bushes a bit, you might get lucky. The American Association for Geriatric Psychiatry has a website (http://www.aagponline.org) at which you can search for its members in your area. You can also call your state psychiatric association. It may have a list of members who are geriatric psychiatrists. If there is a medical school in the area, try calling its department of psychiatry and asking whether there is a geriatric clinic or a faculty member who is a geriatric psychiatrist.

If you find a geriatric psychiatrist who is too far away for regular visits, you might still go for a consultation. It may be well worth driving a few hours for this. You will probably learn a lot and receive recommendations that the professionals who treat you back home can follow. And you'll have more peace of mind.

General Psychiatrists

General, or adult, psychiatrists treat adults of all ages. Some do not accept elderly patients in their practices. Others treat significant numbers of older adults. You can ask how much geriatric work a general psychiatrist does. If older patients make up one-fifth or more of the practice, this may be a good fit for you, especially if you are younger, healthier, and do not take many medications.

If you work with a general psychiatrist, make sure they follow "start low, go slow" with any medication they prescribe for you. Watch out for starting medications at too high a dose, increasing the dose too quickly, or switching too frequently. I have seen many older patients with depression who did not get better despite very active treatment by general psychiatrists. Often they were given ten or more different medications, none of which helped. The problem was that none was tried for longer than one to two weeks, and the doses were too low. I often help such patients by retrying one of the first medications that failed (this takes some convincing, as you might imagine) and gradually increasing the dose to a higher level than was prescribed previously. Voilà! The patient gets better. Patience pays off.

Geriatricians

Geriatricians are primary care physicians who, like geriatric psychiatrists, are specially trained to treat older adults. They are not mental health specialists but are trained to treat depression, and many of them do a fairly good job. Geriatricians are good at recognizing physical factors that contribute to depression. In my experience, many geriatricians do a better job treating geriatric depression than do some general adult psychiatrists. They are less familiar with psychiatry but much more familiar with aging. Unfortunately, geriatricians are also in short supply.

Neurologists

Neurologists specialize in nervous system illnesses, including brain diseases such as Parkinson's and Alzheimer's, so you might think they ought to handle depression, too. Certain neurologists, called behavioral neurologists, are sometimes pretty good at treating depression. But one limitation of neurology practice is that it tends to be consultation oriented. Patients get very thorough evaluations. When I say thorough, believe me, they are. This part is great. Trouble is, what comes next is often not so helpful. I've found that many neurologists prescribe treatment and have you return in six months. It's not that they have no interest in you. It's just that neurologists' practice doesn't allow for regular appointments, which are one of the key ingredients of treating depression.

Nurse Practitioners

Nurse practitioners provide more and more care that only doctors used to do. This varies somewhat state by state. Most nurse practitioners provide primary care. Some states have specialized psychiatric nurse practitioners. Regardless of specialty orientation, few nurse practitioners have training in geriatrics, and they have the same limitations as primary care physicians and general psychiatrists, only with less extensive education and less training.

Psychotherapists

Psychotherapists are most often psychologists or social workers. Some states also allow mental health counselors to practice psychotherapy. If you are lucky, you may be able to find a psychotherapist with geriatric training and experience, but they are even more rare than geriatric psychiatrists. Psychotherapists who have not trained as geriatric specialists may be unfamiliar with the psychological challenges of aging or the psychotherapy approaches and techniques that are most helpful to older adults.

Your primary care doctor may be a good resource for a recommendation to a good therapist. Visiting nurses, directors of senior centers, and case managers at councils on aging may also be familiar with area therapists who are skilled in working with older adults. These people all are in the know, so it's a good sign if the names they give you match up.

WHAT'S IN THE SECRET SAUCE

Wherever you receive treatment for depression, certain characteristics merit the proverbial *Good Housekeeping* seal of approval. Let's go over these so you'll know what to look for.

Hospitality

The setting, such as office, clinic, and so forth, should feel welcoming and receptive to older adults. All personnel, from doctors to receptionists, should communicate well with older adults, in a manner that puts them at ease. There should be sufficient space for walkers, wheelchairs, and entourages of family members. Administrative practices should be accommodating. For example, if you call to make an appointment for your mom, who has Alzheimer's disease, and they require her to make her own appointment, that's probably not the right place.

Care Is Comprehensive and Complex

Medical care is comprehensive when it pays attention not just to the problem at hand but also to all your problems, as well as your list of medications, personal habits, functioning, family situation, and living environment. It is complex when it considers not only all your problems but also how they intertwine and interact. Look for healthcare professionals who see all the moving parts *and* how they fit together.

Family Input

Late-life depression is a family illness. It affects other members of the family. And family input is usually crucial to effective treatment. I think you'll agree that many of the patient stories from earlier chapters illustrated the importance of family. Healthcare services for the elderly should facilitate family input and participation. There are many ways to accomplish this, and all are fine as long as older patients' dignity and privacy are respected.

Continuous Evaluation

You can never take for granted older, frail patients' diagnoses because their conditions can change suddenly and unexpectedly. For example, suppose two weeks after being given a new medication for severe depression you become sluggish, listless, and mildly confused. Members of your family would naturally call the doctor seeking advice. Are you more depressed despite the change? Should the dose be increased? Maybe you are having a bad reaction to the new medication. Rather than raise the dose, maybe it ought to be stopped. How safe is it to make either assumption? Something more serious could be happening. You could be dehydrated or hypoglycemic, or have a urinary tract infection. Or maybe you are in congestive heart failure or have had a stroke. Your family was hoping for advice by phone, but you should expect your doctor to insist that you come to the office or go to the hospital emergency room so that you can be properly reevaluated.

Counseling

Good treatment requires time for counseling. No, not psychotherapy; that's separate. In this context, counseling means talking with patients and their family members about their illnesses and treatments. Good doctors of all specialties do this for all kinds of diseases and treatments. Counseling is crucial in geriatric depression because it is complicated and confusing and older adults have so many concerns. The more your doctor helps you understand your depression and its treatment, the more likely you are to get better.

Tradeoffs Are Carefully Considered and Discussed

What if a very effective treatment for your depression caused you to gain a lot of weight, and that made your diabetes harder to control? How about if it instead made your irritable bowel syndrome worse and gave you even more diarrhea than normal? What if you have chronic kidney disease and there was a 15 percent chance of a treatment worsening your kidney function? Perfect solutions for depression are rare, and such tradeoffs are common in geriatric treatment. Everyone has different values and priorities. Your doctor should help you figure out which tradeoffs fit best with yours.

Expertise with Medications

Each year in the United States, one hundred thousand older adults are hospitalized due to adverse effects of prescribed medications.[6] Some of these incidents are unavoidable. Bad things happen sometimes even with excellent treatment. But in other cases, harmful results can be avoided if medications are prescribed cautiously and wisely. The expertise needed requires being able to anticipate the complex interactions that can occur when older adults take multiple medications for multiple problems.

Here's an example. Let's say you have just begun a medication for depression that can lower your blood pressure and make you light-headed and prone to fall. Your doctor should expect this and take precautions by starting low. But if he or she doesn't know that three other medications you take for various physical conditions also cause blood-pressure-lowering side effects, you could be in trouble. Adding the antidepressant could be the straw that breaks the camel's back. It could make you lightheaded and vulnerable to falling.

Now, imagine that you did fall but were not hurt. Still it was traumatic and you are scared. You blame the new antidepressant and insist on stopping it. But maybe you shouldn't. You'd be back at square one, miserably depressed and more discouraged. What if your doctor had been aware of the common side effects of the other medications and also knew that two of them had substitutes that are free of blood-pressure-lowering side effects? Sticking with the new antidepressant and replacing one or two of the other medications might be a better tradeoff for you. If your doctor sees the big picture and can discuss this type of prescribing complexity with you, you are in good hands.

Time

Treating older adults takes longer. There's no way around it. They have more problems and take more medications than do younger people. Their past histories are longer and their medical records thicker. Doctors must digest scads more information. It can be daunting.

Older adults can also be slow, and depression can make them slower. They move slower. Some think slower. It takes them longer to understand complicated explanations and directions. And, as Irma showed us, older adults experience many reservations about treatment, and it takes time to help them overcome these misgivings. The bottom line is that older adults with depression need more time than is allocated for the average medical appointment; they simply cannot be rushed through.

These days you can't expect doctor visits to feel luxuriously unhurried. And you may feel rushed some of the time. That's unavoidable. But most of the time you should feel there is enough time to cover the most important issues.

HOSPITALIZATION

You might view hospitalization, especially psychiatric hospitalization, as something to be avoided if possible. Most people do. Way back in the last century when I trained, most patients, including older adults, with severe psychiatric problems were initially treated in the hospital. They often stayed weeks or months. This allowed for very thorough and complete treatment. For better or worse, those days are long gone.

The old asylums are also long gone. Nowadays, very few older adults with depression are hospitalized for treatment. The tiny fraction of depressed patients who are include those who can't take care of themselves or are suicidal. Patients still not responding despite prolonged attempts at outpatient treatment are also hospitalized occasionally. These days, hospital stays for psychiatric treatment last only days to a few weeks at most.

Most inpatient geriatric psychiatry treatment occurs in general hospitals on designated psychiatric floors. Many general hospital psychiatric units have specialized geriatric medical-psychiatry programs. A local hospital in your neighborhood might even have one.

I hope that you never need to be hospitalized for treatment of depression. But if you do, it's not the end of the world. A geriatric medical-psychiatry unit might be just what you need. These units are designed for the needs of older adults. They provide integrated medical and psychiatric care, a form of one-stop shopping, which provides fairly comprehensive care. If there is nothing more your primary care physician can do for you, and there are few specialists in your community, then the hospital geriatric medical-psychiatry unit might be the place to get the expertise you need. Hospitalization might be your ticket out of depression, so you should not shun it.

PATIENT EDUCATION

No, you're not going back to school, and there are no tests or grades. But being an educated consumer of health care means you have to know as much as you can about your medical problems, including depression. This is easier said than done.

We live amid an explosion of medical information, but finding information that's helpful to you can be like looking for a needle in a haystack. Information is available everywhere: doctors' offices, hospitals, clinics, senior centers, magazines, books, and the Internet. There's too much, and it's difficult to sift the wheat from the chaff. In my experience, much of the medical information available to the public is too general. It doesn't tell you enough about your situation or answer your individual questions. And much of it is confusing, misleading, or plain wrong.

There's no way around it. At the end of the day, you have to count on your doctors and other healthcare professionals for the information you need. Hopefully they will make sure you understand your condition and its treatment. Just giving you a prescription without taking the time to do this is a recipe for poor treatment.[7] Look for healthcare professionals who take the time to explain things to you.

TREATMENT OF DEPRESSION: A GOLDILOCKS BUSINESS

Another challenge in treating older adults with depression is knowing how much is enough. How far should we push for further improvement? How do we know we're not about to go too far? How do we decide when it's time to settle for good enough, at least for now? When doctors grapple with such questions, that is one sign of good treatment.

As I said earlier, the goal of treating depression should be to help patients feel back to normal. Unfortunately, this is not always achievable. What if the five prior antidepressants you tried didn't work and gave you terrible side effects? And what if the sixth one is working. It agrees with you so far, and you are 60 percent better. Should you press on with further treatment or call it a day and accept 60 percent as good enough? This is a Goldilocks situation. Two types of errors are possible: too much treatment or too little treatment. You want the amount that is just right.

Let's look at the first type of error, too much treatment. You have improved 60 percent, but we do not know whether further improvement is possible. Let's say we decide to increase your treatment, hoping for further improvement, but instead you suffer a terrible side effect and land in the hospital. We should have stayed put and played it safe, and now we regret that we did not.

Now let's look at the second type of error, too little treatment. Suppose a slight increase of medication would make you dramatically better, but we decide to leave well enough alone. You're stuck with a significant amount of depression and missed a chance to get back to normal.

No doctor has a crystal ball that tells him or her what treatment is just right. The art of good treatment is deciding which error, too much treatment or too little treatment, is more important to avoid. Figuring this out involves professional expertise, experience, and judgment, but it also means spending time helping patients and family members understand their choices so they can decide what is best for them.

CONCLUSION

Unless your primary care physician can provide the treatment you need, or you live near a geriatric psychiatry specialist, you will need to make tradeoffs in deciding whom to see for the help you need. Not every older adult with depression gets better, but most do. The odds are in your favor. All you have to do is get started in treatment and stick with it, and remember the five basic rules of thumb:

- Do not accept treatment without a proper and thorough medical evaluation.
- Do not accept treatment without scheduling another appointment fairly soon.
- If you think you have bipolar depression, be wary of antidepressant medications.
- Try to avoid taking benzodiazepines ("benzos").
- Do not sell yourself short. Set your goal to feel back to normal.

I hope this chapter helps you find good treatment and get better. If you do get well, and you get your life back, then I'll be as happy as if I had treated you myself.

NOTES

DEPRESSION IS A LIFE AND DEATH MATTER

1. Martha Bruce et al., "Reducing Suicidal Ideation and Depressive Symptoms in Depressed Older Primary Care Patients," *Journal of the American Medical Association* 291 (2004): 1081–91.

I. OLD AGE IS *NOT* DEPRESSING

1. Lisa C. Barry, "Under-Treatment of Depression in Older Persons," *Journal of Affective Disorders* 136 (2012): 789–96.
2. Robert N. Butler, "Psychiatry and the Elderly: An Overview," *American Journal of Psychiatry* 132 (1975): 893–900.
3. Alzheimer's Association, "2014 Alzheimer's Disease Facts and Figures," *Alzheimer's and Dementia* 10, no. 2 (2014): e47–e92.
4. Melanie Luppa, "Age- and Gender-Specific Prevalence of Depression in Latest-Life: Systematic Review and Meta-Analysis," *Journal of Affective Disorders* 136 (2012): 212–21.
5. Butler, "Psychiatry and the Elderly."
6. Yang Yang, "Social Inequalities in Happiness in the United States, 1972 to 2004: An Age-Period-Cohort Analysis," *American Sociological Review* 73 (2008): 204–26.
7. Daniel Weintraub and Paul E. Ruskin, "Posttraumatic Stress Disorder in the Elderly: A Review," *Harvard Review of Psychiatry* 7 (1999): 144–52.

8. Robert E. Roberts et al., "Does Growing Old Increase the Risk for Depression?" *American Journal of Psychiatry* 154 (1997): 1384–90.

2. WHAT CAUSES DEPRESSION?

1. Sharon Inoye et al., "Geriatric Syndromes: Clinical, Research, and Policy Implications," *Journal of the American Geriatrics Society* 55 (2007): 780–91.

2. Sandra Bell-McGinty et al., "Brain Morphometric Abnormalities in Geriatric Depression: Long-Term Neurobiological Effects of Illness Duration," *American Journal of Psychiatry* 159, no. 8 (2002): 1424–27.

3. Anand Kumar et al., "Frontal White Matter Biochemical Abnormalities in Late-Life Major Depression Detected with Proton Magnetic Resonance Spectroscopy," *American Journal of Psychiatry* 159, no. 4 (2002): 630–36.

4. Howard J. Aizenstein, Carmen Andreescu, and Kathryn L. Edelman, "fMRI Correlates of White Matter Hyperintensities in Late-Life Depression," *American Journal of Psychiatry* 168, no. 10 (2011): 1075–82; Alan Thomas, "Is Depression Really Different in Older People?" *International Psychogeriatrics* 25, no. 11 (November 2013): 1739–42, doi: 101017/S1041610213001038; Eva R. Kenny, "Functional Connectivity in Late-Life Depression Using Resting-State Functional Magnetic Resonance Imaging," *American Journal of Geriatric Psychiatry* 18 (2010): 643–51.

5. Aaron Heller, "Relationships between Changes in Sustained Fronto-Striatal Connectivity and Positive Affect in Major Depression Resulting from Antidepressant Treatment," *American Journal of Psychiatry* 170 (2013): 197–206.

6. Joel R. Sneed, "The Vascular Depression Hypothesis: An Update," *American Journal of Geriatric Psychiatry* 19 (2011): 99–103.

3. DEPRESSION IN OTHER BRAIN DISEASES

1. Louis Kaplan and Iqbal Ahmed, "Depression and Neurological Disease: Their Distinction and Association," *General Hospital Psychiatry* 14 (1992): 177–85.

2. Amane Tateno, Mahito Kimura, and Robert Robertson, "Phenomenological Characteristics of Poststroke Depression," *American Journal of Geriatric Psychiatry* 10 (2002): 575–82.

3. Tateno, Kimura, and Robertson, "Phenomenological Characteristics."

4. Jorge Moncayo Gaete and Julien Bogousslavsky, "Post-Stroke Depression," *Expert Review of Neurotherapeutics* 8, no. 1 (2008): 75–92, doi: 10.1586/14737175.8.1.758.1.

5. George Zubenko et al., "A Collaborative Study of the Emergence and Clinical Features of the Major Depression Syndrome of Alzheimer's Disease," *American Journal of Psychiatry* 160 (2003): 857–66.

6. Roseanne DeFronzo Dobkin et al., "Depression in Parkinson's Disease: Symptom Improvement and Residual Symptoms after Acute Pharmacologic Management," *American Journal of Geriatric Psychiatry* 19 (2011): 222–29.

7. Theresa Zesiewicz et al., "Current Issues in Depression in Parkinson's Disease," *American Journal of Geriatric Psychiatry* 7 (1999): 110–18.

8. Thomas Ehmann et al., "Depressive Symptoms in Parkinson's Disease: A Comparison with Disabled Control Subjects," *Journal of Geriatric Psychiatry and Neurology* 2 (1989): 3–9.

9. Jeffrey Cummings, "Depression and Parkinson's Disease: A Review," *American Journal of Psychiatry* 149 (1992): 443–54.

4. WHAT'S IN A NAME?

1. *Diagnostic and Statistical Manual of Mental Disorders*, 5th ed. (Washington, DC: American Psychiatric Association, 2013), 155–88.

2. "Major Depression and the 'Bereavement Exclusion,'" American Psychiatric Association, accessed December 13, 2014, http://www.dsm5.org.

3. "Beat the Winter Blues," National Institute of Health, *News in Health* (January 2013), accessed December 18, 2014, http://newsinhealth.nih.gov.

4. Joseph J. Gallo et al., "Depression without Sadness: Functional Outcomes of Nondysphoric Depression in Later Life," *Journal of the American Geriatrics Society* 45 (1997): 570–78.

5. Robert M. Rohrbaugh, Alan P. Siegal, and Earl L. Giller, "Irritability as a Symptom of Depression in the Elderly," *Journal of the American Geriatrics Society* 1988 (36): 736–38.

6. George S. Alexopoulos et al., "Clinical Presentation of the 'Depression-Executive Dysfunction Syndrome' of Late Life," *American Journal of Geriatric Psychiatry* 10, no. 1 (2002): 98–106.

5. "WHAT YOU DON'T KNOW WON'T HURT YOU"

1. Peter D. Kramer, *Against Depression* (New York: Viking Penguin, 2005), xii.
2. Floriana S. Luppino et al., "Overweight, Obesity, and Depression," *Archives of General Psychiatry* 67 (2010): 220–29.
3. Yael Harris and James K. Cooper, "Depressive Symptoms in Older People Predict Nursing Home Admission," *Journal of the American Geriatrics Society* 54 (2006): 593–97.
4. Brenda W. J. Pennix et al., "Depressive Symptoms and Physical Decline in Community-Dwelling Older Adults," *Journal of the American Medical Association* 279 (1998): 1720–26.
5. Owen M. Wolkowitz, Victor I. Reus, and Synthia H. Mellon, "Of Sound Mind and Body: Depression, Disease, and Accelerated Aging," *Dialogues in Clinical Neuroscience* 13, no. 1 (2011): 25–39.
6. Brian E. Leonard, "Stress, Depression and the Immune System," *Stress Medicine* 16, no. 3 (2000): 133–37.
7. Ilan S. Wittstein et al., "Neurohumoral Features of Myocardia Stunning Due to Sudden Emotional Stress," *New England Journal of Medicine* 352 (2005): 539–48.
8. Wolkowitz, Reus, and Mellon, "Of Sound Mind and Body"; Brandon Chad McKinney and Etienne Sibille, "The Age-by-Disease Interaction Hypothesis of Late-Life Depression," *American Journal of Geriatric Psychiatry* 21 (2013): 418–32; Josine E. Verhoeven et al., "Major Depressive Disorder and Accelerated Cellular Aging: Results from a Large Psychiatric Cohort Study," *Molecular Psychiatry* 19, no. 8 (August 2014): 895–901, accessed November 12, 2013, doi: 10.1038/mp.2013.151.
9. Wolkowitz, Reus, and Mellon, "Of Sound Mind and Body."

6. WHEN HEARTACHE CAUSES HEART "ACHE"

1. Centers for Disease Control and Prevention, Division for Heart Disease and Stroke Prevention, accessed January 15, 2015, http://www.CDC.gov.
2. Marijke A. Bremmer et al., "Depression in Older Age Is a Risk Factor for First Ischemic Cardiac Events," *American Journal of Geriatric Psychiatry* 14 (2006): 523–30.

3. Jessica M. Brown et al., "Risk of Coronary Heart Disease Events over 15 Years among Older Adults with Depressive Symptoms," *American Journal of Geriatric Psychiatry* 19 (2011): 721–29.

4. Jeanine Romanelli et al., "The Significance of Depression in Older Patients after Myocardial Infarction," *Journal of the American Geriatrics Society* 50 (2002): 817–22.

5. Judith Lichtman et al., "Depression as a Risk Factor for Poor Prognosis among Patients with Acute Coronary Syndrome: Systematic Review and Recommendations," *Circulation* 129 (2014): 1350–69.

6. Hendrika J. Luijendijk et al., "Heart Failure and Incident Late-Life Depression," *Journal of the American Geriatrics Society* 58 (2010): 1441–46.

7. Mary A. Whooly et al., "Depressive Symptoms, Health Behaviors, and Risk of Cardiovascular Events in Patients with Coronary Heart Disease," *Journal of the American Medical Association* 300 (2008): 2379–88.

8. Martin Samuels, "The Brain-Heart Connection," *Circulation* 116 (2007): 77–84; Robert M. Carney et al., "Major Depression, Heart Rate, and Plasma Norepinephrine in Patients with Coronary Heart Disease," *Biological Psychiatry* 45, no. 4 (1999): 458–63.

9. Wittstein et al., "Neurohumoral Features."

10. Alexander H. Glassman and J. Thomas Bigger Jr., "Antidepressants in Coronary Heart Disease: SSRIs Reduce Depression, But Do They Save Lives?" *Journal of the American Medical Association* 297, no. 4 (2007): 411–12.

11. Robert M. Carney and Kenneth E. Freedland, "Treatment-Resistant Depression and Mortality after Acute Coronary Syndrome," *American Journal of Psychiatry* 166 (2009): 410–17; Peter de Jonge et al., "Nonresponse to Treatment for Depression following Myocardial Infarction: Association with Subsequent Cardiac Events," *American Journal of Psychiatry* 164 (2007): 1371–78.

7. TREATMENT OF DEPRESSION MAY BE A STROKE OF LUCK

1. Centers for Disease Control and Prevention, "Stroke Facts," accessed January 25, 2015, http://www.cdc.gov.

2. National Stroke Association, "Understand Stroke," accessed January 25, 2015, http://www.stroke.org.

3. Jia-Yi Dong et al., "Depression and Risk of Stroke," *Stroke* 43 (2012): 32–37; Caroline Jackson and Gita Mishra, "Depression and Risk of Stroke in Middle Aged Women," *Stroke* 44 (2014): 1555–60; An Pan et al., "Depression and Risk of Stroke Morbidity and Mortality," *Journal of the American Medical Association* 306 (2011): 1241–49.

4. Jackson and Mishra, "Depression and Risk of Stroke."

5. Henry Brodaty et al., "Rates of Depression at 3 and 15 Months Post-stroke and Their Relationship with Cognitive Decline: The Sydney Stroke Study," *American Journal of Geriatric Psychiatry* 15 (2007): 477–86.

6. National Stroke Association, "Preventing Another Stroke," accessed January 29, 2015, http://www.stroke.org.

7. Gerli Sibolt et al., "Post-Stroke Depression and Depression-Executive Dysfunction Syndrome Are Associated with Recurrence of Ischemic Stroke," *Cerebrovascular Diseases* 36 (2013): 336–43.

8. Jesse Stewart, Anthony J. Perkins, and Christopher M. Callahan, "Effect of Collaborative Care for Depression on Risk of Cardiovascular Events: Data from the IMPACT Randomized Controlled Trial," *Psychosomatic Medicine* 76 (2014): 29–37.

9. Yan Chen et al., "Treatment Effects of Antidepressants in Patients with Post-Stroke Depression: A Meta-Analysis," *Annals of Pharmacotherapy* 40 (2006): 2115–22.

10. Ricardo E. Jorge et al., "Escitalopram and Enhancement of Cognitive Recovery Following Stroke," *Archives of General Psychiatry* 67 (2010): 187–96; Gillian E. Mead, Cheng-Fang Hsieh, and Maree Hackett, "Selective Serotonin Reuptake Inhibitors for Stroke Recovery," *Journal of the American Medical Association* 310 (2013): 1066–67.

8. DEPRESSION AND DIABETES

1. Antonio Campayo et al., "Depressive Disorder and Incident Diabetes Mellitus: The Effect of Characteristics of Depression," *American Journal of Psychiatry* 167 (2010): 580–88.

2. Wayne J. Katon, "The Comorbidity of Diabetes Mellitus and Depression," *American Journal of Medicine* 121 (2008): S8–S15.

3. Patrick J. Lustman and Ray E. Clouse, "Depression in Diabetic Patients: The Relationship between Mood and Glycemic Control," *Journal of Diabetes and Its Complications* 19 (2005): 113–22.

4. Andrew H. Ford et al., "Insulin Resistance and Depressive Symptoms in Older Men: The Health in Men Study," *American Journal of Psychiatry* 23, no. 8 (2015): 872–80.

5. Katon, "Comorbidity of Diabetes."

6. Lustman and Clouse, "Depression in Diabetic Patients."

7. Marjolein M. Iversen et al., "Is Depression a Risk Factor for Diabetic Foot Ulcers? 11-Year Follow-up of the Nord-Trondelag Health Study (HUNT)," *Journal of Diabetes and Its Complications* 20 (2015): 20–25.

8. Lindsay B. Kimbro et al., "Depression and All-Cause Mortality in Persons with Diabetes Mellitus: Are Older Adults at Higher Risk? Results from the Translating Research into Action for Diabetes Study," *Journal of the American Geriatrics Society* 62 (2014): 1017–22.

9. Katon, "Comorbidity of Diabetes."

10. American Diabetes Association, "Depression," accessed February 2, 2015, http://www.diabetes.org.

11. Patrick J. Lustman et al., "Sertraline for Prevention of Depression Recurrence in Diabetes Mellitus," *Archives of General Psychiatry* 63 (2006): 521–29.

12. Hillary R. Bogner et al., "Diabetes, Depression and Death," *Diabetes Care* 30 (2007): 3005–10.

13. Katon, "Comorbidity of Diabetes."

14. Jennifer McSharry et al., "The Chicken and Egg Thing: Cognitive Representations and Self-Management of Multimorbidity in People with Diabetes and Depression," *Psychology and Health* 28 (2013): 103–19.

15. American Diabetes Association, "Standards of Medical Care in Diabetes: 2007," *Diabetes Care* 30 (2007): S4–S41.

9. BREATHE EASIER

1. Centers for Disease Control and Prevention, "Chronic Obstructive Pulmonary Disease (COPD)," accessed February 9, 2015, http://www.cdc.gov/copd/index.htm.

2. American Lung Association, "Chronic Obstructive Pulmonary Disease Fact Sheet," accessed February 9, 2015, http://www.lung.org.

3. Evan Atlantis et al., "Bidirectional Associations between Clinically Relevant Depression or Anxiety and COPD," *Chest* 144 (2013): 766–77.

4. Atlantis et al., "Bidirectional Associations"; Marc Maravitlles et al., "Factors Associated with Depression and Severe Depression in Patients with COPD," *Respiratory Medicine* 108 (2014): 1615–25.

5. Maravitlles et al., "Factors Associated with Depression."

6. Neil Jordan et al., "Effect of Depression Care on Outcomes in COPD Patients with Depression," *Chest* 135 (2009): 626–32.

7. Coen H. van Gool et al., "Relationship between Changes in Depressive Symptoms and Unhealthy Lifestyles in Late Middle Aged and Older Persons: Results from the Longitudinal Aging Study Amsterdam," *Age and Ageing* 32 (2003): 81–87.

8. D. A. Grosneberg et al., "Neurogenic Mechanisms in Bronchial Inflammatory Disease," *Allergy* 59 (2004): 1139–52; George I. Viamontes and

Charles B. Nemeroff, "The Physiologic Effect of Mental Processes on Major Body Systems," *Psychiatric Annals* 40 (2010): 367–80.

9. Osama M. Momtaz et al., "Effect of Treatment of Depression and Anxiety on Physiological State of Severe COPD Patients," *Egyptian Journal of Chest Diseases and Tuberculosis* 64, no. 1 (January 2015): 29–34, accessed February 9, 2015, http://dx.doi.org/10.1016/j.ejcdt.2014.08.006; George S. Alexopoulos et al., "Untangling Therapeutic Ingredients of a Personalized Intervention for Patients with Depression and Severe COPD," *American Journal of Psychiatry* 22 (2014): 1316–24.

10. Jingjing Qian et al., "Effects of Depression Diagnosis and Antidepressant Treatment on Mortality in Medicare Beneficiaries with Chronic Obstructive Pulmonary Disease," *Journal of the American Geriatrics Society* 61 (2013): 754–61.

11. Abebaw M. Yohannes, Martin Connolly, and Robert C. Baldwin, "A Feasibility Study of Antidepressant Drug Therapy in Depressed Elderly Patients with Chronic Obstructive Pulmonary Disease," *International Journal of Geriatric Psychiatry* 16 (2001): 451–54.

12. George S. Alexopoulos et al., "Outcomes of Depressed Patients Undergoing Inpatient Pulmonary Rehabilitation," *American Journal of Geriatric Psychiatry* 14 (2006): 466–75.

10. DEPRESSION AND CHRONIC KIDNEY DISEASE

1. S. Susan Heyadati, Venkata Yalamanchili, and Frederic O. Finkelstein, "A Practical Approach to the Treatment of Depression in Patients with Chronic Kidney Disease and End-Stage Renal Disease," *Kidney International* 81 (2012): 247–55.

2. Quinn D. Kellerman et al., "Association between Depressive Symptoms and Mortality Risk in Chronic Kidney Disease," *Health Psychology* 29 (2010): 594–600.

3. Heyadati, Yalamanchili, and Finkelstein, "Practical Approach."

4. Liang Feng, Keng Bee Yap, and Tze Pin Ng, "Depressive Symptoms in Older Adults with Chronic Kidney Disease: Mortality, Quality of Life Outcomes, and Correlates," *American Journal of Geriatric Psychiatry* 21, no. 6 (2013): 570–79; S. Susan Heyadati et al., "Association between Major Depressive Disorder Episodes in Patients with Chronic Kidney Disease and Initiation of Dialysis, Hospitalization, or Death," *Journal of the American Medical Association* 303 (2010): 1946–53.

5. Kellerman et al., "Association between Depressive Symptoms and Mortality Risk."

6. Feng, Yap, and Ng, "Depressive Symptoms."

7. Heyadati, Yalamanchili, and Finkelstein, "Practical Approach"; Heyadati et al., "Association between Major Depressive Disorder Episodes."

8. Baris Afsar, "The Relationship of Serum Cortisol Levels with Depression, Cognitive Function and Sleep Disorders in Chronic Kidney Disease and Hemodialysis Patients," *Psychiatry Quarterly* 85 (2014): 479–86.

9. Mohammad Taraz, Saeideh Taraz, and Simin Dashti-Khavidaki, "Association between Depression and Inflammatory/Anti-inflammatory Cytokines in Chronic Kidney Disease and End-Stage Renal Disease Patients: A Review of Literature," *Hemodialysis International* 19 (2015): 11–22.

10. Kellerman et al., "Association between Depressive Symptoms and Mortality Risk."

11. Kellerman et al., "Association between Depressive Symptoms"; Dora Zalai, Lilla Szeifert, and Marta Novak, "Psychological Distress and Depression in Patients with Chronic Kidney Disease," *Seminars in Dialysis* 4 (2012): 428–38.

12. Heyadati, Yalamanchili, and Finkelstein, "Practical Approach"; Zalai, Szeifert, and Novak, "Psychological Distress."

13. Heyadati, Yalamanchili, and Finkelstein, "Practical Approach."

14. National Kidney Foundation, "Dialysis: Deciding to Stop," accessed February 21, 2015, https://www.kidney.org.

11. DEPRESSION AND CANCER

1. William F. Pirl et al., "Depression and Survival in Metastatic Non-Small-Cell Lung Cancer: Effects of Early Palliative Care," *Journal of Clinical Oncology* 30 (2012): 1310–15; Oscar Arrieta et al., "Association of Depression and Anxiety in Quality of Life, Treatment Adherence, and Prognosis in Patients with Advanced Non-small Cell Lung Cancer," *Annals of Surgical Oncology* 20 (2013): 1941–48.

2. M. Sharpe et al., "Major Depression in Outpatients Attending a Regional Cancer Centre: Screening and Unmet Treatment Needs," *British Journal of Cancer* 90 (2004): 314–20.

3. Campbell S. Roxburgh and Donald C. McMillan, "Cancer and Systemic Inflammation: Treat the Tumour and Treat the Host," *British Journal of Cancer* 110, no. 6 (2014): 1409–12.

4. Roxburgh and McMillan, "Cancer and Systemic Inflammation."

5. Michel Reich, "Depression and Cancer: Recent Data on Clinical Issues, Research Challenges, and Treatment Approaches," *Current Opinion in Oncology* 20 (2008): 353–59.

6. Yi-Hua Chen and Herng-Ching Lin, "Increased Risk of Cancer Subsequent to Severe Depression: A Nationwide Population-Based Study," *Journal of Affective Disorders* 131 (2011): 200–206.

7. Chen and Lin, "Increased Risk of Cancer."

8. M. Pinquart and P.R. Duberstein, "Depression and Cancer Mortality: A Meta-Analysis," *Psychological Medicine* 40 (2010): 1797–1810.

9. Jillian R. Satlin, Wolfgang Linden, and Melanie J. Phillips, "Depression as a Predictor of Disease Progression and Mortality in Cancer Patients," *Cancer* 115 (2009): 5349–61.

10. Ibid.

11. Janine Giese-David et al., "Decrease in Depression Symptoms Is Associated with Longer Survival in Patients with Metastatic Breast Cancer: A Secondary Analysis," *Journal of Clinical Oncology* 29 (2011): 413–20.

12. World Health Association, "Cancer: Fact Sheet," last updated February 2015, accessed February 27, 2015, http://www.who.int.

13. Ravishanka Jayadevappa et al., "The Burden of Depression in Prostate Cancer," *Psycho-Oncology* 21 (2012): 1338–45.

14. Casey A. Boyd et al., "The Effect of Depression on Stage at Diagnosis, Treatment, and Survival in Pancreatic Adenocarcinoma," *Surgery* 152 (2012): 403–13.

15. Pirl et al., "Depression and Survival."

16. James S. Goodwin, Dong D. Zhang, and Glenn V. Ostir, "Effect of Depression on Diagnosis, Treatment, and Survival of Older Women with Breast Cancer," *Journal of the American Geriatrics Society* 52 (2004): 106–11.

17. Satlin, Linden, and Phillips, "Depression as a Predictor."

18. Anthony B. Miller et al., "Twenty-Five-Year Follow-up for Breast Cancer Incidence and Mortality of the Canadian National Breast Screening Study: Randomized Screening Trial," *British Medical Journal* 348 (2014): g366. doi: 10.1136/bmj.g366.

19. Goodwin, Zhang, and Ostir, "Effect of Depression."

20. Arrieta et al., "Association of Depression and Anxiety."

21. Boyd et al., "Effect of Depression"; Goodwin, Zhang, and Ostir, "Effect of Depression."

22. Pinquart and Duberstein, "Depression and Cancer Mortality."

23. Boyd et al., "Effect of Depression"; Marco Colleoni et al., "Depression and Degree of Acceptance of Adjuvant Cytotoxic Drugs," *Lancet* 356 (2000): 1326–27.

24. Barbara Given and Charles Given, "Older Adults and Cancer Treatment." *Cancer* 113, suppl. 12 (2008): 3505–11.

25. Arrieta et al., "Association of Depression and Anxiety."

26. Arrieta et al., "Association of Depression and Anxiety"; Roxburgh and McMillan, "Cancer and Systemic Inflammation."

27. Given and Given, "Older Adults."

28. Reich, "Depression and Cancer."

12. DEPRESSION AND ARTHRITIS

1. Elizabeth H. B. Lin, "Depression and Osteoarthritis," *American Journal of Medicine* 121 (2008): S16–S19.

2. Elizabeth H. B. Lin et al., "Effect of Improving Depression Care on Pain and Functional Outcomes among Older Adults with Arthritis," *Journal of the American Medical Association* 290 (2003): 2428–34.

3. Linda P. Fried et al., "Diagnosis of Illness Presentation in the Elderly," *Journal of the American Geriatrics Society* 39 (1991): 117–23.

4. Travis O. Bruce, "Comorbid Depression in Rheumatoid Arthritis: Pathophysiology and Clinical Implications," *Current Psychiatry Reports* 10 (2008): 258–64.

5. Alex J. Zautra, Mary C. David, and John W. Reich, "Comparison of Cognitive Behavioral and Mindfulness Meditation Interventions on Adaptation to Rheumatoid Arthritis for Patients With and Without History of Recurrent Depression," *Journal of Consulting and Clinical Psychology* 76 (2008): 408–21.

6. Zautra, David, and Reich, "Comparison of Cognitive Behavioral."

7. Bruce, "Comorbid Depression."

13. DEPRESSION AND PARKINSON'S DISEASE

1. Cheng-Che Shen et al., "Risk of Parkinson Disease after Depression," *Neurology* 81 (2013): 1538–44.

2. Shen et al., "Risk of Parkinson Disease."

3. Shen et al., "Risk of Parkinson Disease."

4. Theresa Zesiewicz et al., "Current Issues in Depression in Parkinson's Disease," *American Journal of Geriatric Psychiatry* 7, no. 2 (1999): 110–18.

5. Zesiewicz et al., "Current Issues in Depression in Parkinson's Disease."

6. Irene Hegeman Richard and Roger Kurlan, "The Under-Recognition of Depression in Parkinson's Disease," *Neuropsychiatric Disease and Treatment* 2 (2006): 349–53.

7. C. Allyson Jones, Sheri L. Pohar, and Scott B. Patten, "Major Depression and Health-Related Quality of Life in Parkinson's Disease," *General Hospital Psychiatry* 31 (2009): 334–40.

8. Jones, Pohar, and Patten, "Major Depression."

9. Richard and Kurlan, "Under-Recognition of Depression."

10. Roseanne D. Dobkin et al., "Cognitive-Behavioral Therapy for Depression in Parkinson's Disease: A Randomized, Controlled Trial," *American Journal of Psychiatry* 168 (2011): 1066–74.

11. Claudio Franceschi et al., "Inflamm-Aging," *Annals of the New York Academy of Science* 908 (2000): 244–54.

12. Ann M. Hemmerle, James P. Herman, and Kim B. Seroogy, "Stress, Depression, and Parkinson's Disease," *Experimental Neurology* 233 (2012): 79–86.

13. Hemmerle, Herman, and Seroogy, "Stress, Depression, and Parkinson's Disease."

14. DEPRESSION AND ALZHEIMER'S DISEASE

1. Amy L. Byers and Kristine Yaffe, "Depression and Risk for Developing Dementia," *Nature Reviews Neurology* 7 (2011): 323–31.

2. Maria Shriver, "A Woman's Nation Takes On Alzheimer's," in "The Shriver Report: A Study by Maria Shriver and the Alzheimer's Association," accessed March 21, 2015, http://www.alz.org.

3. Yuan Gao et al., "Depression as a Risk Factor for Dementia and Mild Cognitive Impairment: A Meta-Analysis of Longitudinal Studies," *International Journal of Geriatric Psychiatry* 28 (2013): 441–49.

4. Byers and Yaffe, "Depression and Risk"; Patricia Gracia-García et al., "Depression and Incident Alzheimer Disease: The Impact of Disease Severity," *American Journal of Geriatric Psychiatry* 23, no. 2 (2015): 119–29; Deborah E. Barnes et al., "Midlife vs. Late-Life Depressive Symptoms and Risk of Dementia," *Archives of General Psychiatry* 69 (2012): 493–98; Vonetta M. Dotson, May A. Beydoun, and Alan B. Zonderman, "Recurrent Depressive Symptoms and the Incidence of Dementia and Mild Cognitive Impairment," *Neurology* 75 (2010): 27–34.

5. Hajime Baba et al., "Metabolism of Amyloid-B Protein May Be Affected in Depression." *Journal of Clinical Psychiatry* 73 (2012): 115–20.

6. Gracia-García et al., "Depression and Incident Alzheimer Disease."

7. Shriver, "Woman's Nation."

8. Anton Porsteinsson and Inga M. Antonsdottir, "Depression and Risk of Dementia: Exploring the Interface," *Journal of Clinical Psychiatry* 74 (2013): 1262–63.

15. DEPRESSION CAN BE A REAL PAIN: DEPRESSION AND PAIN

1. Graziano Onder et al., "Association between Pain and Depression among Older Adults in Europe: Results from the Aged in Home Care (Ad-HOC) Project: A Cross-Sectional Study," *Journal of Clinical Psychiatry* 66 (2005): 982–88.

2. Linn-Heidi Lunde and Inger Hilde Nordhus, "The Effectiveness of Cognitive and Behavioral Treatment of Chronic Pain in the Elderly: A Quantitative Review," *Journal of Clinical Psychology in Medical Settings* 16 (2009): 254–62.

3. Dennis C. Turk, Akiko Okifuji, and Lisa Scharff, "Chronic Pain and Depression: Role of Perceived Impact and Perceived Control in Different Age Cohorts," *Pain* 61 (1995): 93–101.

4. Lunde and Nordhus, "Effectiveness of Cognitive and Behavioral Treatment."

5. Elizabeth H. B. Lin et al., "Effect of Improving Depression Care on Pain and Functional Outcomes among Older Adults with Arthritis," *Journal of the American Medical Association* 290 (2003): 2428–34.

6. Martin D. Cheatle, "Depression, Chronic Pain, and Suicide by Overdose: On the Edge," *Pain Medicine* 12 (2011): S43–S48.

7. Cheatle, "Depression, Chronic Pain, and Suicide."

8. M. Carrington Reid et al., "Depressive Symptoms as a Risk Factor for Disabling Back Pain in Community-Dwelling Older Persons," *Journal of the American Geriatrics Society* 51 (2003): 1710–17.

9. David W. Swanson, "Chronic Pain as a Third Pathologic Emotion," *American Journal of Psychiatry* 141 (1984): 210–14; Dennis C. Turk and Peter Salovey, "Chronic Pain as a Variant of Depressive Disease," *Journal of Nervous and Mental Disease* 172 (1984): 398–407.

10. Changsu Han and Chi-Un Pae, "Pain and Depression: A Neurobiological Perspective of Their Relationship," *Psychiatry Investigations* 12 (2015): 1–8.

11. Ana Miriam Velly et al., "The Effect of Catastrophizing and Depression on Chronic Pain: A Prospective Cohort Study of Temporomandibular Muscle and Joint Pain Disorders," *Pain* 152 (2011): 2377–83.

12. Turk, Okifuji, and Scharff, "Chronic Pain and Depression."

13. Velly et al., "Effect of Catastrophizing."

14. Katherine A. Raichle, Joan M. Romano, and Mark P. Jensen, "Partner Responses to Patient Pain and Well Behaviors and Their Relationship to Patient Pain Behavior, Functioning, and Depression," *Pain* 152 (2011): 82–88.

15. Lin et al., "Effect of Improving."

16. Lunde and Nordhus, "Effectiveness of Cognitive and Behavioral Treatment."

16. DON'T TAKE THE FALL FOR DEPRESSION: DEPRESSION AND FALLING

1. Andrea Iaboni and Alastair Flint, "The Complex Interplay of Depression and Falls in Older Adults: A Clinical Review," *American Journal of Geriatric Psychiatry* 21 (2013): 484–92.

2. Sébastien Grenier et al., "Depressive Symptoms Are Independently Associated with Recurrent Falls in Community-Dwelling Older Adults," *International Psychogeriatrics* 26, no. 9 (2014): 1511–20, doi: 10.1017/S104161021400074X.

3. Talia Herman et al., "Executive Control Deficits as a Prodrome to Falls in Healthy Older Adults: A Prospective Study Linking Thinking, Walking, and Falling," *Journals of Gerontology: A Biological Science Medical Science* 65A (2010): 1086–92.

4. Tasha Kvelde et al., "Depressive Symptomatology as a Risk Factor for Falls in Older People: Systematic Review and Meta-Analysis," *Journal of the American Geriatrics Society* 61 (2013): 694–706; Lien Quach et al., "Depression, Antidepressants, and Falls among Community-Dwelling Elderly People: The MOBILIZE Boston Study," *Journals of Gerontology: A Biological Science Medical Science* 68 (2013): 1575–81.

5. Iaboni and Flint, "Complex Interplay of Depression and Falls."

6. Tamar C. Brandler et al., "Depressive Symptoms and Gait Dysfunction in the Elderly," *American Journal of Geriatric Psychiatry* 20 (2012): 425–32.

7. Jolanda C. M. van Haastregt et al., "Feelings of Anxiety and Symptoms of Depression in Community-Living Older Persons Who Avoid Activity for Fear of Falling," *American Journal of Geriatric Psychiatry* 16 (2008): 186–93.

8. Mooyeon Oh-Park et al., "Transient versus Persistent Fear of Falling in Community-Dwelling Older Adults: Incidence and Risk Factors," *Journal of the American Geriatrics Society* 59 (2011): 1225–31.

9. Nandini Deshpande et al., "Activity Restriction Induced by Fear of Falling and Objective and Subjective Measures of Physical Function: A Pros-

pective Cohort Study," *Journal of the American Geriatrics Society* 56 (2008): 615–20.

10. Iaboni and Flint, "Complex Interplay of Depression and Falls."

11. Iaboni and Flint, "Complex Interplay of Depression and Falls"; G. A. Rixt Zilstra et al., "Interventions to Reduce Fear of Falling in Community-Living Older People: A Systematic Review," *Journal of the American Geriatrics Society* 55 (2007): 603–15.

17. "YOU CAN LEAD A HORSE TO WATER . . ."

1. Yohannes, Connolly, and Baldwin, "Feasibility Study."

2. Yohannes, Connolly, and Baldwin, "Feasibility Study."

18. YOU'RE NEVER TOO OLD

1. Barnett S. Meyers, "Treatment and Course of Geriatric Depression," *American Journal of Geriatric Psychiatry* 10 (2002): 497–502; J. Craig Nelson, Kevin L. Delucchi, and Lon S. Schneider, "Moderators of Outcome in Late-Life Depression: A Patient-Level Meta-Analysis," *American Journal of Psychiatry* 170 (2013): 651–59; Charles F. Reynolds III et al., "Treatment of 70+-Year-Olds with Recurrent Major Depression: Excellent Short-Term but Brittle Long-Term Response," *American Journal of Geriatric Psychiatry* 7 (1999): 64–69.

2. Patricia Patricio et al., "Differential and Converging Molecular Mechanism of Antidepressants' Action in the Hippocampal Dentate Gyrus," *Neuropsychopharmacology* 40 (2015): 339–49; Larry W. Thompson et al., "Comparison of Desipramine and Cognitive/Behavioral Therapy in the Treatment of Elderly Outpatients with Mild-to-Moderate Depression," *American Journal of Geriatric Psychiatry* 9 (2001): 225–40.

3. Thompson et al., "Comparison of Desipramine."

4. Philippe Landreville et al., "Older Adults' Acceptance of Psychological and Pharmacological Treatments for Depression," *Journal of Gerontology* 56B (2001): 285–91.

5. Ritsaert Lieverse et al., "Bright Light Treatment in Elderly Patients with Nonseasonal Major Depressive Disorder," *Archives of General Psychiatry* 68 (2011): 61–70.

6. Philip D. Sloane, Mariana Figueiro, and Lauren Cohen, "Light as Therapy for Sleep Disorders and Depression in Older Adults," *Clinical Geriatrics* 16, no. 3 (2008): 25–31.

7. Roumen Milev et al., "Repetitive Transcranial Magnetic Stimulation for Treatment of Medication-Resistant Depression in Older Adults," *Journal of ECT* 25 (2009): 44–49.

8. Heller, "Relationships between Changes."

9. Reynolds et al., "Treatment of 70+-Year-Olds."

10. Charles F. Reynolds III et al., "Which Elderly Patients with Remitted Depression Remain Well with Continued Interpersonal Psychotherapy after Discontinuation of Antidepressant Medication?" *American Journal of Psychiatry* 154 (1997): 958–62.

19. WHEN LIFE GIVES YOU LEMONS, MAKE LEMONADE

1. Eric J. Lenze et al., "Incomplete Response in Late-Life Depression: Getting to Remission," *Dialogues in Clinical Neuroscience* 10 (2008): 419–30.

2. Patricio et al., "Differential and Converging."

3. J. Craig Nelson, Kevin Delucchi, and Lon Schneider, "Suicidal Thinking and Behavior during Treatment with Sertraline in Late-Life Depression," *American Journal of Geriatric Psychiatry* 15 (2007): 573–80.

4. Centers for Disease Control and Prevention, "Adults and Older Adult Adverse Drug Events," accessed May 22, 2015, http://www.cdc.gov.

5. Munir Pirmohamed et al., "Adverse Drug Reactions as Cause of Admission to Hospital: Prospective Analysis of 18,820 Patients," *British Medical Journal* 329 (2004): 15–19; Anne Benard-Laribi et al., "Incidence of Hospital Admissions Due to Adverse Drug Reactions in France: The EMIR Study," *Fundamental and Clinical Pharmacology* 29 (2015): 106–11.

20. LIFESTYLE PRACTICES, HERBAL TREATMENTS, AND NUTRITIONAL SUPPLEMENTS

1. Jose Ness et al., "Use of Complementary Medicine in Older Americans: Results from the Health and Retirement Study," *Gerontologist* 45 (2005): 516–24; Geraldine Moses, "Complementary and Alternative Medicine Use in the Elderly," *Journal of Pharmacology Practice and Research* 35 (2005): 63–68.

2. National Center for Complementary and Integrative Health, "Complementary, Alternative, or Integrative Health: What's in a Name?" October 2008, accessed April 29, 2015, https://nccih.nih.gov.

3. Marlene P. Freeman, "Omega-3 Fatty Acids in Major Depressive Disorder," *Journal of Clinical Psychiatry* 7, suppl. 5 (2009): 7–11.

4. Freeman, "Omega-3 Fatty Acids."

5. Joseph Bergman et al., "Curcumin as an Add-On to Antidepressant Treatment: A Randomized, Double-Blind, Placebo-Controlled Pilot Clinical Study," *Clinical Neuropharmacology* 36 (2013): 73–77.

6. Bergman et al., "Curcumin as an Add-On."

7. Freeman, "Omega-3 Fatty Acids."

8. Bergman et al., "Curcumin as an Add-On."

9. J. Craig Nelson, "S-Adenosyl Methionine (SAMe) Augmentation in Major Depression," *American Journal of Psychiatry* 167 (2010): 889–91.

10. George I. Papakostas et al., "S-Adenosyl Methionine (SAMe) Augmentation for Serotonin Reuptake Inhibitors for Antidepressant Nonresponders with Major Depressive Disorder: A Double-Blind, Randomized Clinical Trial," *American Journal of Psychiatry* 167 (2010): 942–48.

11. J. Craig Nelson, "The Evolving Story of Folate in Depression and the Therapeutic Potential of L-Methylfolate," *American Journal of Psychiatry* 169 (2012): 1223–25.

12. Richard C. Shelton, "St. John's Wort (Hypericum Perforatum) in Major Depression," *Journal of Clinical Psychiatry* 70, suppl. 5 (2009): 23–27.

13. Gary Cooney, Kerry Dwan, and Gillian Mead, "Exercise for Depression," *Journal of the American Medical Association* 311 (2014): 2432–33.

14. Carol Palmer, "Exercise as a Treatment for Depression in Elders," *Clinical Practice* 17 (2005): 60–66.

15. Kripalu Center for Yoga and Health, "What Is Yoga?" accessed May 3, 2015, http://www.kripalu.org.

16. Holger Cramer et al., "Yoga for Depression: A Systematic Review and Meta-Analysis," *Depression and Anxiety* 30 (2013): 1068–83.

17. Michael R. Irwin and Richard Olmstead, "Mitigating Cellular Inflammation in Older Adults: A Randomized Controlled Trial of Tai Chi Chih," *American Journal of Geriatric Psychiatry* 20 (2012): 764–72.

18. Peter M. Wayne et al., "Effect of Tai Chi on Cognitive Performance in Older Adults: Systematic Review and Meta-Analysis," *Journal of the American Geriatrics Society* 62 (2014): 25–39.

19. Helen Lavretsky et al., "Complementary Use of Tai Chi Chih Augments Escitalopram Treatment of Geriatric Depression: A Randomized Controlled Trial," *American Journal of Geriatric Psychiatry* 19, no. 10 (2011): 839–50.

20. "Acupuncture," Mayo Clinic, accessed April 29, 2015, http://www. mayoclinic.org.

21. Junmei Wu et al., "Acupuncture for Depression: A Review of Clinical Applications," *Canadian Journal of Psychiatry* 57, no. 7 (2012): 397–405.

22. Sylvia Schroer et al., "Acupuncture for Depression: Exploring Model Validity and the Related Issue of Credibility in the Context of Designing a Pragmatic Trial," *CNS Neurosciences and Therapeutics* 18, no. 4 (2012): 318–26; Hugh MacPherson et al., "Acupuncture for Depression: Patterns of Diagnosis and Treatment within a Randomised Controlled Trial," *Evidence-Based Complementary and Alternative Medicine* (2013): 1–9.

23. Deborah Bowden, Lorna Goddard, and John Gruzelier, "A Randomised Controlled Single-Blind Trial of the Efficacy of Reiki at Benefitting Mood and Well-Being," *Evidence-Based Complementary and Alternative Medicine* 8 (2011): 1–8, doi: 10.1155/2011381862.

24. Moses, "Complementary and Alternative Medicine."

22. THE SHOCKING FACTS ABOUT SHOCK TREATMENT

1. Karen G. Kelly and Marc Zisselman, "Update on Electroconvulsive Therapy (ECT) in Older Adults," *Journal of the American Geriatrics Society* 48 (2000): 560–66.

2. Maayanit Sigler, Dov Aizenberg, and Abraham Weizman, "Continuation and Maintenance Electroconvulsive Therapy in Elderly Depressed Patients," *International Journal of Geriatric Psychopharmacology* 1, no. 4 (1998): 205–7.

3. Tracy A. Tomac et al., "Safety and Efficacy of Electroconvulsive Therapy in Patients over Age 85," *American Journal of Geriatric Psychiatry* 5 (1997): 126–30.

4. Carl Salzman, Eileen Wong, and B. Cody Wright, "Drug and ECT Treatment of Depression in the Elderly 1996–2001: A Literature Review," *Biological Psychiatry* 52 (2002): 265–84.

5. Tomac et al., "Safety and Efficacy of Electroconvulsive Therapy."

23. GETTING THE TREATMENT YOU NEED

1. Christopher M. Callahan, "Quality Improvement Research on Late Life Depression in Primary Care," *Medical Care* 39 (2001): 772–84.

2. Institute of Medicine of the National Academies, "The Mental Health and Substance Use Workforce for Older Adults: In Whose Hands" (Washington, DC: National Academies Press, 2012).

3. M. Tai-Seale et al., "Two-Minute Mental Health Care for Elderly Patients: Inside Primary Care Visits," *Journal of the American Geriatrics Society* 55 (2007): 1903–11.

4. Callahan, "Quality Improvement Research."

5. Carmen Andreescu et al., "Empirically Derived Decision Trees for the Treatment of Late-Life Depression," *American Journal of Psychiatry* 165 (2008): 855–62.

6. Centers for Disease Control and Prevention, "Adults and Older Adult Adverse Drug Events."

7. Yohannes, Connolly, and Baldwin, "Feasibility Study."

BIBLIOGRAPHY

Afsar, Baris. "The Relationship of Serum Cortisol Levels with Depression, Cognitive Function and Sleep Disorders in Chronic Kidney Disease and Hemodialysis Patients." *Psychiatry Quarterly* 85 (2014): 479–86.

Aizenstein, Howard J., Carmen Andreescu, and Kathryn L. Edelman. "fMRI Correlates of White Matter Hyperintensities in Late-Life Depression." *American Journal of Psychiatry* 168, no. 10 (2011): 1075–82.

Alexopoulos, George S., Dimitri N. Kiosses, Sibel Klimstra, Balkrishna Kalayam, and Martha L. Bruce. "Clinical Presentation of the 'Depression-Executive Dysfunction Syndrome' of Late Life." *American Journal of Geriatric Psychiatry* 10, no. 1 (2002): 98–106.

Alexopoulos, George S., Dimitris N. Kiosses, Jo Anne Sirey, Dora Kanellopoulos, Joanna K. Seirup, Richard S. Novitch, Samiran Ghosh, Samprit Banerjee, and Patrick J. Raue. "Untangling Therapeutic Ingredients of a Personalized Intervention for Patients with Depression and Severe COPD." *American Journal of Psychiatry* 22 (2014): 1316–24.

Alexopoulos, George S., Jo Anne Sirey, Patrick J. Raue, Dora Kanellopoulos, Timothy E. Clark, and Richard S. Novitch. "Outcomes of Depressed Patients Undergoing Inpatient Pulmonary Rehabilitation." *American Journal of Geriatric Psychiatry* 14 (2006): 466–75.

Alzheimer's Association. "2014 Alzheimer's Disease Facts and Figures." *Alzheimer's and Dementia* 10, no. 2 (2014): e47–e92.

American Diabetes Association. "Depression." Accessed February 2, 2015. http://www.diabetes.org.

———. "Standards of Medical Care in Diabetes: 2007." *Diabetes Care* 30 (2007): S4–S41.

American Lung Association. "Chronic Obstructive Pulmonary Disease Fact Sheet." Accessed February 9, 2015. http://www.lung.org.

American Psychiatric Association. *Diagnostic and Statistical Manual of Mental Disorders*. 5th ed. Washington, DC: Author, 2013.

———. "Major Depression and the 'Bereavement Exclusion.'" Accessed December 13, 2014. http://www.dsm5.org.

Andreescu, Carmen, Benoit H. Mulsant, Patricia R. Houck, Ellen M. Whyte, Sati Mazumdar, Alexandre Y. Dombrovski, Bruce G. Pollock, and Charles F. Reynolds. "Empirically Derived Decision Trees for the Treatment of Late-Life Depression." *American Journal of Psychiatry* 165 (2008): 855–62.

Arrieta, Oscar, Laura P. Angulo, Carolina Nunez-Valencia, Yuzmiren Dorantes-Gallareta, Eleazar O. Macedo, Dulce Martinez-Lopez, Salvador Alvarado, Jose-Francisco Corona-Cruz, and Luis F. Onate-Ocana. "Association of Depression and Anxiety in Quality of Life, Treatment Adherence, and Prognosis in Patients with Advanced Non-small Cell Lung Cancer." *Annals of Surgical Oncology* 20 (2013): 1941–48.

Atlantis, Evan, Paul Fahey, Belinda Cochrance, and Sheree Smith. "Bidirectional Associations between Clinically Relevant Depression or Anxiety and COPD." *Chest* 144 (2013): 766–77.

Baba, Hajime, Yoshiyuki Nakano, Hitoshi Maeshima, Emi Satomura, Yohei Kita, Toshihito Suzuki, and Heil Arai. "Metabolism of Amyloid-B Protein May Be Affected in Depression." *Journal of Clinical Psychiatry* 73 (2012): 115–20.

Barnes, Deborah E., Kristine Yaffe, Amy Byers, Mark McCormick, Catherine Schaefer, and Rachel A. Whitmer. "Midlife vs Late-Life Depressive Symptoms and Risk of Dementia." *Archives of General Psychiatry* 69 (2012): 493–98.

Barry, Lisa C. "Under-Treatment of Depression in Older Persons." *Journal of Affective Disorders* 136 (2012): 789–96.

Bell-McGinty, Sandra, Meryl A. Butters, Carolyn Cidis Meltzer, Phil J. Greer, Charles F. Reynolds III, and James T. Becker. "Brain Morphometric Abnormalities in Geriatric Depression: Long-Term Neurobiological Effects of Illness Duration." *American Journal of Psychiatry* 159, no. 8 (2002): 1424–27.

Benard-Laribi, Anne, Ghada Miremont-Salam, Marie-Christine Perault-Pochat, Pernelle Noize, and Francoise Haramburu. "Incidence of Hospital Admissions Due to Adverse Drug Reactions in France: The EMIR Study." *Fundamental and Clinical Pharmacology* 29 (2015): 106–11.

Bergman, Joseph, Chanoch Miodownik, Yuly Bersudsky, Shmuel Sokolik, Paul P. Lerner, Anatoly Kreinin, Jacob Polakiewicz, and Vladimir Lerner. "Curcumin as an Add-On to Antidepressant Treatment: A Randomized, Double-Blind, Placebo-Controlled Pilot Clinical Study." *Clinical Neuropharmacology* 36 (2013): 73–77.

Bogner, Hillary R., Edward P. Post, Knashawn H. Morales, and Martha L. Bruce. "Diabetes, Depression and Death." *Diabetes Care* 30 (2007): 3005–10.

Bowden, Deborah, Lorna Goddard, and John Gruzelier. "A Randomised Controlled Single-Blind Trial of the Efficacy of Reiki at Benefitting Mood and Well-Being." *Evidence-Based Complementary and Alternative Medicine* 8 (2011): 1–8. doi: 10.1155/2011381862.

Boyd, Casey A., Jaime Benarroch-Gampel, Kristin M. Shefield, Yimel Han, Yong-Fang Kuo, and Taylor S. Riall. "The Effect of Depression on Stage at Diagnosis, Treatment, and Survival in Pancreatic Adenocarcinoma." *Surgery* 152 (2012): 403–13.

Brandler, Tamar C., Cuiling Wang, Mooyeon Oh-Park, Roee Holtzer, and Joe Verghese. "Depressive Symptoms and Gait Dysfunction in the Elderly." *American Journal of Geriatric Psychiatry* 20 (2012): 425–32.

Bremmer, Marijke A., Witte J. G. Hoogendijk, Dorly J. H. Deeg, Robert A. Schoevers, Bianca W. M. Schalk, and Aartjan T. F. Beekman. "Depression in Older Age Is a Risk Factor for First Ischemic Cardiac Events." *American Journal of Geriatric Psychiatry* 14 (2006): 523–30.

Brodaty, Henry, Adrienne Withall, Annette Altendorf, and Perminder S. Sachdev. "Rates of Depression at 3 and 15 Months Poststroke and Their Relationship with Cognitive Decline: The Sydney Stroke Study." *American Journal of Geriatric Psychiatry* 15 (2007): 477–86.

Brown, Jessica M., Jesse C. Stewart, Timothy E. Stump, and Christopher M. Callahan. "Risk of Coronary Heart Disease Events over 15 Years among Older Adults with Depressive Symptoms." *American Journal of Geriatric Psychiatry* 19 (2011): 721–29.

Bruce, Martha, Thomas R. Ten Have, Charles F. Reynolds III, Ira I. Katz, Herbert C. Schulberg, Benoit H. Mulsant, Gregory K. Brown, Gail J. McAvay, Jane L. Pearson, and George S. Alexopoulos. "Reducing Suicidal Ideation and Depressive Symptoms in Depressed Older Primary Care Patients." *Journal of the American Medical Association* 291 (2004): 1081–91.

Bruce, Travis O. "Comorbid Depression in Rheumatoid Arthritis: Pathophysiology and Clinical Implications." *Current Psychiatry Reports* 10 (2008): 258–64.

Butler, Robert N. "Psychiatry and the Elderly: An Overview." *American Journal of Psychiatry* 132 (1975): 893–900.

Byers, Amy L., and Kristine Yaffe. "Depression and Risk for Developing Dementia." *Nature Reviews Neurology* 7 (2011): 323–31.

Callahan, Christopher M. "Quality Improvement Research on Late Life Depression in Primary Care." *Medical Care* 39 (2001): 772–84.

Campayo, Antonio, Peter de Jonge, Juan F. Roy, Pedro Saz, Concepcion de la Camara, Miguel A. Quintanilla, Guillermo Marcos, Javier Santabarbara, and Antonio Lobo. "Depressive Disorder and Incident Diabetes Mellitus: The Effect of Characteristics of Depression." *American Journal of Psychiatry* 167 (2010): 580–88.

Carney, Robert M., and Kenneth E. Freedland. "Treatment-Resistant Depression and Mortality after Acute Coronary Syndrome." *American Journal of Psychiatry* 166 (2009): 410–17.

Carney, Robert M., Kenneth E. Freedland, Richard C. Veith, Philip E. Cryer, Judith A. Skala, Tiffany Lynch, and Allan S. Jaffe. "Major Depression, Heart Rate, and Plasma Norepinephrine in Patients with Coronary Heart Disease." *Biological Psychiatry* 45, no. 4 (1999): 458–63.

Centers for Disease Control and Prevention. "Adults and Older Adult Adverse Drug Events." Accessed May 22, 2015. http://www.cdc.gov.

———. "Chronic Obstructive Pulmonary Disease (COPD)." Accessed February 9, 2015. http://www.cdc.gov/copd/index.htm.

———. "Stroke Facts." Accessed January 25, 2015. http://www.cdc.gov.

Cheatle, Martin D. "Depression, Chronic Pain, and Suicide by Overdose: On the Edge." *Pain Medicine* 12 (2011): S43–S48.

Chen, Yan, Jeff J. Guo, Slyan Zhan, and Nick C. Patel. "Treatment Effects of Antidepressants in Patients with Post-Stroke Depression: A Meta-Analysis." *Annals of Pharmacotherapy* 40 (2006): 2115–22.

Chen, Yi-Hua, and Herng-Ching Lin. "Increased Risk of Cancer Subsequent to Severe Depression: A Nationwide Population-Based Study." *Journal of Affective Disorders* 131 (2011): 200–206.

Colleoni, Marco, Marlo Mandale, Glulia Peruzzotti, Chris Robertson, Anne Bredart, and Aron Goldhirsch. "Depression and Degree of Acceptance of Adjuvant Cytotoxic Drugs." *Lancet* 356 (2000): 1326–27.

Cooney, Gary, Kerry Dwan, and Gillian Mead. "Exercise for Depression." *Journal of the American Medical Association* 311 (2014): 2432–33.

Cramer, Holger, Romy Lauche, Jost Langhorst, and Gustav Dobos. "Yoga for Depression: A Systematic Review and Meta-Analysis." *Depression and Anxiety* 30 (2013): 1068–83.

Cummings, Jeffrey. "Depression and Parkinson's Disease: A Review." *American Journal of Psychiatry* 149 (1992): 443–54.

de Jonge, Peter, Adriaan Honig, Joost P. van Melle, Aart H. Schene, Astrid M. G. Kuyper, Dorien Tulner, Annique Schins, and Johan Ormel. "Nonresponse to Treatment for Depression Following Myocardial Infarction: Association with Subsequent Cardiac Events." *American Journal of Psychiatry* 164 (2007): 1371–78.

Deshpande, Nandini, E. Jeffrey Metter, Fulvio Lauretani, Stefania Bandinelli, Jack Guralnik, and Luigi Ferrucci. "Activity Restriction Induced by Fear of Falling and Objective and Subjective Measures of Physical Function: A Prospective Cohort Study." *Journal of the American Geriatrics Society* 56 (2008): 615–20.

Dobkin, Roseanne D., Matthew Menza, Lesley A. Allen, Michael A. Gara, Margery H. Mark, Jade Tiu, Karina L. Bienfait, and Jill Friedman. "Cognitive-Behavioral Therapy for Depression in Parkinson's Disease: A Randomized, Controlled Trial." *American Journal of Psychiatry* 168 (2011): 1066–74.

Dobkin, Roseanne DeFronzo, Matthew Menza, Karina L. Bienfait, Michael Gara, Humberto Marin, Margery H. Mark, Allison Dicke, and Jill Friedman. "Depression in Parkinson's Disease: Symptom Improvement and Residual Symptoms after Acute Pharmacologic Management." *American Journal of Geriatric Psychiatry* 19 (2011): 222–29.

Dong, Jia-Yi, Yong-Hong Zhang, Jian Tong, and LiQuang Qin. "Depression and Risk of Stroke." *Stroke* 43 (2012): 32–37.

Dotson, Vonetta M., May A. Beydoun, and Alan B. Zonderman. "Recurrent Depressive Symptoms and the Incidence of Dementia and Mild Cognitive Impairment." *Neurology* 75 (2010): 27–34.

Ehmann, Thomas, Richard J. Beninger, Merek J. Gawel, and Richard J. Riopelle. "Depressive Symptoms in Parkinson's Disease: A Comparison with Disabled Control Subjects." *Journal of Geriatric Psychiatry and Neurology* 2 (1989): 3–9.

Feng, Liang, Keng Bee Yap, and Tze Pin Ng. "Depressive Symptoms in Older Adults with Chronic Kidney Disease: Mortality, Quality of Life Outcomes, and Correlates." *American Journal of Geriatric Psychiatry* 21, no. 6 (2013): 570–79.

Ford, Andrew H., Leon Flicker, Graeme J. Hankey, Bu B. Yeap, S. A. Paul Chubb, Jonathan Golledge, and Osvaldo P. Almeida. "Insulin Resistance and Depressive Symptoms in Older Men: The Health in Men Study." *American Journal of Psychiatry* 23, no. 8 (2015): 872–80.

Franceschi, Claudio, Massimilliano Bonafe, Silvan Valensin, Fabiola Olivier, Maria DeLuca, Enzo Ottaviani, and Giovanna DeBenedictis. "Inflamm-Aging." *Annals of the New York Academy of Science* 908 (2000): 244–54.

Freeman, Marlene P. "Omega-3 Fatty Acids in Major Depressive Disorder." *Journal of Clinical Psychiatry* 7, suppl. 5 (2009): 7–11.

Fried, Linda P., Dean J. Storer, Deborah E. King, and Frances Lodder. "Diagnosis of Illness Presentation in the Elderly." *Journal of the American Geriatrics Society* 39 (1991): 117–23.

Gaete, Jorge Moncayo, and Julien Bogousslavsky. "Post-stroke Depression." *Expert Review of Neurotherapeutics* 8, no. 1 (2008): 75–92. doi: 10.1586/14737175.8.1.758.1.

Gallo, Joseph J., Peter V. Rabins, Constantine G. Lyketsos, Allen Y. Tien, and James C. Anthony. "Depression without Sadness: Functional Outcomes of Nondysphoric Depression in Later Life." *Journal of the American Geriatrics Society* 45 (1997): 570–78.

Gao, Yuan, Changquan Huang, Kexiang Zhao, Ouyan Ma, Xuan Qui, Lei Zhang, Yun Xiu, Lin Chen, Wei Lu, Chunxia Huang, Yong Tang, and Qian Xiao. "Depression as a Risk Factor for Dementia and Mild Cognitive Impairment: A Meta-Analysis of Longitudinal Studies." *International Journal of Geriatric Psychiatry* 28 (2013): 441–49.

Giese-David, Janine, Kate Collie, Kate M. S. Rancourt, Eric Neri, Helena C. Kraemer, and David Spiegel. "Decrease in Depression Symptoms Is Associated with Longer Survival in Patients with Metastatic Breast Cancer: A Secondary Analysis." *Journal of Clinical Oncology* 29 (2011): 413–20.

Given, Barbara, and Charles Given. "Older Adults and Cancer Treatment." *Cancer* 113, suppl. 12 (2008): 3505–11.

Glassman, Alexander H., and J. Thomas Bigger Jr. "Antidepressants in Coronary Heart Disease: SSRIs Reduce Depression, But Do They Save Lives?" *Journal of the American Medical Association* 297, no. 4 (2007): 411–12.

Goodwin, James S., Dong D. Zhang, and Glenn V. Ostir. "Effect of Depression on Diagnosis, Treatment, and Survival of Older Women with Breast Cancer." *Journal of the American Geriatrics Society* 52 (2004): 106–11.

Gracia-García, Patricia, Concepcion de la Camara, Javier Santabarbara, Raul Lopez-Anton, Miguel Angel Quintanilla, Tirso Ventura, Guilerma Marcos, Antonio Campayo, Pedro Saz, Constantine Lyketsos, and Antonio Lobo. "Depression and Incident Alzheimer Disease: The Impact of Disease Severity." *American Journal of Geriatric Psychiatry* 23, no. 2 (2015): 119–29.

Grenier, Sébastien, Marie-Christine Payette, Francis Langlois, Thien Tuong, and Louis Bherer. "Depressive Symptoms Are Independently Associated with Recurrent Falls in Community-Dwelling Older Adults." *International Psychogeriatrics* 26, no. 9 (2014): 1511–20. doi: 10.1017/S104161021400074X.

Grosneberg, D. A., D. Quarcoo, N. Frossard, and A. Fisher. "Neurogenic Mechanisms in Bronchial Inflammatory Disease." *Allergy* 59 (2004): 1139–52.

Han, Changsu, and Chi-Un Pae. "Pain and Depression: A Neurobiological Perspective of Their Relationship." *Psychiatry Investigations* 12 (2015): 1–8.

Harris, Yael, and James K. Cooper. "Depressive Symptoms in Older People Predict Nursing Home Admission." *Journal of the American Geriatrics Society* 54 (2006): 593–97.

Hegeman Richard, Irene, and Roger Kurlan. "The Under-Recognition of Depression in Parkinson's Disease." *Neuropsychiatric Disease and Treatment* 2 (2006): 349–53.

Hemmerle, Ann M., James P. Herman, and Kim B. Seroogy. "Stress, Depression, and Parkinson's Disease." *Experimental Neurology* 233 (2012): 79–86.

Heller, Aaron. "Relationships between Changes in Sustained Fronto-Striatal Connectivity and Positive Affect in Major Depression Resulting from Antidepressant Treatment." *American Journal of Psychiatry* 170 (2013): 197–206.

Herman, Talia, Anat Mirelman, Nir Giladi, Avraham Schweiger, and Jeffrey M. Hausdorff. "Executive Control Deficits as a Prodrome to Falls in Healthy Older Adults: A Prospective Study Linking Thinking, Walking, and Falling." *Journals of Gerontology: A Biological Science Medical Science* 65A (2010): 1086–92.

Heyadati, S. Susan, Abu T. Minhujjudin, Masoud Afshar, Robert D. Tota, Madhykar H. Trivedi, and A. John Rush. "Association between Major Depressive Disorder Episodes in Patients with Chronic Kidney Disease and Initiation of Dialysis, Hospitalization, or Death." *Journal of the American Medical Association* 303 (2010): 1946–53.

Heyadati, S. Susan, Venkata Yalamanchili, and Frederic O. Finkelstein. "A Practical Approach to the Treatment of Depression in Patients with Chronic Kidney Disease and End-Stage Renal Disease." *Kidney International* 81 (2012): 247–55.

Iaboni, Andrea, and Alastair Flint. "The Complex Interplay of Depression and Falls in Older Adults: A Clinical Review." *American Journal of Geriatric Psychiatry* 21 (2013): 484–92.

Inoye, Sharon, Stephanie Studenski, Mary Tinetti, and George A. Kuchel. "Geriatric Syndromes: Clinical, Research, and Policy Implications." *Journal of the American Geriatrics Society* 55 (2007): 780–91.

Institute of Medicine of the National Academies. "The Mental Health and Substance Use Workforce for Older Adults: In Whose Hands." Washington, DC: National Academies Press, 2012.

Irwin, Michael R., and Richard Olmstead. "Mitigating Cellular Inflammation in Older Adults: A Randomized Controlled Trial of Tai Chi Chih." *American Journal of Geriatric Psychiatry* 20 (2012): 764–72.

Iversen, Marjolein M., Grethe S. Tell, Birgitte Espehaug, Kristian Midthjell, Marit Graue, Berit Rokne, Line Iden Berge, and Truls Osbye. "Is Depression a Risk Factor for Diabetic Foot Ulcers? 11-Year Follow-up of the Nord-Trondelag Health Study (HUNT)." *Journal of Diabetes and Its Complications* 20 (2015): 20–25.

Jackson, Caroline, and Gita Mishra. "Depression and Risk of Stroke in Middle Aged Women." *Stroke* 44 (2014): 1555–60.

Jayadevappa, Ravishanka, S. Bruce Malkowicz, Sumedha Chhatre, Jerry C. Johnson, and Joseph J. Gallo. "The Burden of Depression in Prostate Cancer." *Psycho-Oncology* 21 (2012): 1338–45.

Jones, C. Allyson, Sheri L. Pohar, and Scott B. Patten. "Major Depression and Health-Related Quality of Life in Parkinson's Disease." *General Hospital Psychiatry* 31 (2009): 334–40.

Jordan, Neil, Todd A. Lee, Marcia Valenstein, Paul A. Pirraglia, and Keven B. Weiss. "Effect of Depression Care on Outcomes in COPD Patients with Depression." *Chest* 135 (2009): 626–32.

Jorge, Ricardo E., Laura Acion, David Moser, Harold P. Adams, and Robert G. Robinson. "Escitalopram and Enhancement of Cognitive Recovery Following Stroke." *Archives of General Psychiatry* 67 (2010): 187–96.

Kaplan, Louis, and Iqbal Ahmed. "Depression and Neurological Disease: Their Distinction and Association." *General Hospital Psychiatry* 14 (1992): 177–85.

Katon, Wayne J. "The Comorbidity of Diabetes Mellitus and Depression." *American Journal of Medicine* 121 (2008): S8–S15.

Kellerman, Quinn D., Alan J. Christensen, Austin S. Baldwin, and William J. Lawton. "Association between Depressive Symptoms and Mortality Risk in Chronic Kidney Disease." *Health Psychology* 29 (2010): 594–600.

Kelly, Karen G., and Marc Zisselman. "Update on Electroconvulsive Therapy (ECT) in Older Adults." *Journal of the American Geriatrics Society* 48 (2000): 560–66.

Kenny, Eva R. "Functional Connectivity in Late-Life Depression Using Resting-State Functional Magnetic Resonance Imaging." *American Journal of Geriatric Psychiatry* 18 (2010): 643–51.

Kimbro, Lindsay B., Carol M. Mangione, W. Neil Steers, O. Kenrik Duru, Laura McEwan, Andrew Karter, and Susan L. Ettner. "Depression and All-Cause Mortality in Persons with Diabetes Mellitus: Are Older Adults at Higher Risk? Results from the Translating Research into Action for Diabetes Study." *Journal of the American Geriatrics Society* 62 (2014): 1017–22.

Kramer, Peter D. *Against Depression.* New York: Viking Penguin, 2005.

Kripalu Center for Yoga and Health. "What Is Yoga?" Accessed May 3, 2015. http://www.kripalu.org.

Kumar, Anand, Thomas Albert, Helen Lavretsky, Kenneth Yue, Amir Huda, John Curran, Talaignair Venkatraman, Lavern Estanol, Jim Mintz, Michael Mega, and Arthur Toga. "Frontal White Matter Biochemical Abnormalities in Late-Life Major Depression Detected with Proton Magnetic Resonance Spectroscopy." *American Journal of Psychiatry* 159, no. 4 (2002): 630–36.

Kvelde, Tasha, Catherine McVeigh, Barbara Toson, Mark Greenaway, Stephen R. Lord, Kim Delbaere, and Jacqueline C. T. Close. "Depressive Symptomatology as a Risk Factor for Falls in Older People: Systematic Review and Meta-Analysis." *Journal of the American Geriatrics Society* 61 (2013): 694–706.

Landreville, Philippe, Julie Landry, Lucie Bailargeon, Anne Guerette, and Evelyn Matteau. "Older Adults' Acceptance of Psychological and Pharmacological Treatments for Depression." *Journal of Gerontology* 56B (2001): 285–91.

Lavretsky, Helen, Lily L. Alstein, Richard E. Olmstead, Linda M. Ercoli, Marguertie Riparetti-Brown, Natalie St. Cyr, and Michael R. Irwin. "Complementary Use of Tai Chi Chih Augments Escitalopram Treatment of Geriatric Depression: A Randomized Controlled Trial." *American Journal of Geriatric Psychiatry* 19, no. 10 (2011): 839–50.

Lenze, Eric J., Meera Sheffrin, Henry C. Driscoll, Benoit H. Mulsant, Bruce G. Pollack, Mary Amanda Dew, Frank Lotrich, Bernie Devlin, Robert Bies, and Charles F. Reynolds III. "Incomplete Response in Late-Life Depression: Getting to Remission." *Dialogues in Clinical Neuroscience* 10 (2008): 419–30.

Leonard, Brian E. "Stress, Depression and the Immune System." *Stress Medicine* 16, no. 3 (2000): 133–37.

Lichtman, Judith, Erika S. Foelicher, James A. Blumenthal, Robert M. Carney, Lynn V. Doering, Nancy Frasure-Smith, Kenneth E. Freeland, Allan S. Jaffe, Erica C. Leifheit-Limson, David S. Sheps, Viola Viccarino, and Lawson Wulsin. "Depression as a Risk Factor for Poor Prognosis among Patients with Acute Coronary Syndrome: Systematic Review and Recommendations." *Circulation* 129 (2014): 1350–69.

Lieverse, Ritsaert, Marjan M. A. Nielen, Dick J. Veltman, Bernard M. J. Uitdehaag, Eus J. W. van Someren, Jan H. Smit, and Witte J. G. Hoogendijk. "Bright Light Treatment in Elderly Patients with Nonseasonal Major Depressive Disorder." *Archives of General Psychiatry* 68 (2011): 61–70.

Lin, Elizabeth H. B. "Depression and Osteoarthritis." *American Journal of Medicine* 121 (2008): S16–S19.

Lin, Elizabeth H. B., Wayne Katon, Michael Von Korff, Lingqi Tang, John W. Williams, Kurt Kroenke, Enid Hunkeler, Linda Harpole, Mark Hegel, Patricia Arean, Marc Hoffing, Richard Della Penna, Chris Langston, and Jurgen Unutzer. "Effect of Improving Depression Care on Pain and Functional Outcomes among Older Adults with Arthritis." *Journal of the American Medical Association* 290 (2003): 2428–34.

Luijendijk, Hendrika J., Henning Tiemeier, Julia F. van den Berg, Gysele S. Bleumink, Albert Hofman, and Bruno H. C. Stricker. "Heart Failure and Incident Late-Life Depression." *Journal of the American Geriatrics Society* 58 (2010): 1441–46.

Lunde, Linn-Heidi, and Inger Hilde Nordhus. "The Effectiveness of Cognitive and Behavioral Treatment of Chronic Pain in the Elderly: A Quantitative Review." *Journal of Clinical Psychology in Medical Settings* 16 (2009): 254–62.

Luppa, Melanie. "Age- and Gender-Specific Prevalence of Depression in Latest-Life: Systematic Review and Meta-Analysis." *Journal of Affective Disorders* 136 (2012): 212–21.

Luppino, Floriana S., Leonore M. de Wit, Paul F. Bouvy, Theo Stijnen, Pim Cuijpers, Brenda W. J. H. Pennix, and Frans G. Zitman. "Overweight, Obesity, and Depression." *Archives of General Psychiatry* 67 (2010): 220–29.

Lustman, Patrick J., and Ray E. Clouse. "Depression in Diabetic Patients: The Relationship between Mood and Glycemic Control." *Journal of Diabetes and Its Complications* 19 (2005): 113–22.

Lustman, Patrick J., Ray E. Clouse, Billy D. Nix, Kenneth E. Freedland, Eugene H. Rubin, Janet B. McGill, Monique M. Williams, Alan J. Gelenberg, Paul S. Ciechanowski, and Irl B. Hirsch. "Sertraline for Prevention of Depression Recurrence in Diabetes Mellitus." *Archives of General Psychiatry* 63 (2006): 521–29.

Maravitlles, Marc, Jesus Molina, Jose Antonio Quintano, Anna Campuzano, Joselin Perez, and Carlos Roncero. "Factors Associated with Depression and Severe Depression in Patients with COPD." *Respiratory Medicine* 108 (2014): 1615–25.

Mayo Clinic. "Acupuncture." Accessed April 29, 2015. http://www.mayoclinic.org.

McKinney, Brandon Chad, and Etienne Sibille. "The Age-by-Disease Interaction Hypothesis of Late-Life Depression." *American Journal of Geriatric Psychiatry* 21 (2013): 418–32.

MacPherson, Hugh, Ben Elliot, Ann Hopton, Harriet Lansdown, and Stewart Richmond. "Acupuncture for Depression: Patterns of Diagnosis and Treatment within a Randomised Controlled Trial." *Evidence-Based Complementary and Alternative Medicine* (2013): 1–9.

McSharry, Jennifer, Felicity L. Bishop, Rona Moss-Morris, and Tony Kendrick. "The Chicken and Egg Thing: Cognitive Representations and Self-Management of Multimorbidity in People with Diabetes and Depression." *Psychology and Health* 28 (2013): 103–19.

Mead, Gillian E., Cheng-Fang Hsieh, and Maree Hackett. "Selective Serotonin Reuptake Inhibitors for Stroke Recovery." *Journal of the American Medical Association* 310 (2013): 1066–67.

Meyers, Barnett S. "Treatment and Course of Geriatric Depression." *American Journal of Geriatric Psychiatry* 10 (2002): 497–502.

Milev, Roumen, Gaby Abraham, Gary Hasey, and Jason Lee Cabaj. "Repetitive Transcranial Magnetic Stimulation for Treatment of Medication-Resistant Depression in Older Adults." *Journal of ECT* 25 (2009): 44–49.

Miller, Anthony B., Claus Wall, Cornelia J. Baines, Ping Sun, Teresa To, and Steven A. Narod. "Twenty-Five-Year Follow-up for Breast Cancer Incidence and Mortality of the Canadian National Breast Screening Study: Randomized Screening Trial." *British Medical Journal* 348 (2014): g366. doi: 10.1136/bmj.g366.

Momtaz, Osama M., Salwa M. Rabei, Nezar R. Tawfike, and Ali A. Hasan. "Effect of Treatment of Depression and Anxiety on Physiological State of Severe COPD Patients." *Egyptian Journal of Chest Diseases and Tuberculosis* 64, no. 1 (January 2015): 29–34. Accessed February 9, 2015. http://dx.doi.org/10.1016/j.ejcdt.2014.08.006.

Moses, Geraldine. "Complementary and Alternative Medicine Use in the Elderly." *Journal of Pharmacology Practice and Research* 35 (2005): 63–68.

National Center for Complementary and Integrative Health. "Complementary, Alternative, or Integrative Health: What's in a Name?" October 2008. Accessed April 29, 2015. https://nccih.nih.gov.

National Institute of Health. "Beat the Winter Blues." *News in Health* (January 2013). Accessed December 18, 2014. http://newsinhealth.nih.gov.

National Kidney Foundation. "Dialysis: Deciding to Stop." Accessed February 21, 2015. https://www.kidney.org.

National Stroke Association. "Preventing Another Stroke." Accessed January 29, 2015. http://www.stroke.org.

———. "Understand Stroke." Accessed January 25, 2015. http://www.stroke.org.

Nelson, J. Craig. "The Evolving Story of Folate in Depression and the Therapeutic Potential of L-Methylfolate." *American Journal of Psychiatry* 169 (2012): 1223–25.

———. "S-Adenosyl Methionine (SAMe) Augmentation in Major Depression." *American Journal of Psychiatry* 167 (2010): 889–91.

Nelson, J. Craig, Kevin Delucchi, and Lon Schneider. "Suicidal Thinking and Behavior during Treatment with Sertraline in Late-Life Depression." *American Journal of Geriatric Psychiatry* 15 (2007): 573–80.

Nelson, J. Craig, Kevin L. Delucchi, and Lon S. Schneider. "Moderators of Outcome in Late-Life Depression: A Patient-Level Meta-Analysis." *American Journal of Psychiatry* 170 (2013): 651–59.

Ness, Jose, Dominic J. Cirillo, David R. Weir, Nicole L. Nisly, and Robert B. Wallace. "Use of Complementary Medicine in Older Americans: Results from the Health and Retirement Study." *Gerontologist* 45 (2005): 516–24.

Oh-Park, Mooyeon, Xiaonan Xue, Roee Holtzer, and Joe Verghese. "Transient versus Persistent Fear of Falling in Community-Dwelling Older Adults: Incidence and Risk Factors." *Journal of the American Geriatrics Society* 59 (2011): 1225–31.

Onder, Graziano, Francesco Landi, Giovanni Gambassi, Rosa Liperoti, Manuel Soldato, Chiara Catanti, Harriet Fine-Soveri, Cornelius Katona, Iain Carpenter, and Roberto Bernabei. "Association between Pain and Depression among Older Adults in Europe: Results from the Aged in Home Care (AdHOC) Project: A Cross-Sectional Study." *Journal of Clinical Psychiatry* 66 (2005): 982–88.

Palmer, Carol. "Exercise as a Treatment for Depression in Elders." *Clinical Practice* 17 (2005): 60–66.

Pan, An, Qi Sun, Olvia I. Okereke, Kathryn M. Rexrode, and Frank B. Hu. "Depression and Risk of Stroke Morbidity and Mortality." *Journal of the American Medical Association* 306 (2011): 1241–49.

Papakostas, George I., David Mischoulon, Irene Shyu, Jonathan E. Alpert, and Maurizio Fava. "S-Adenosyl Methionine (SAMe) Augmentation for Serotonin Reuptake Inhibitors for Antidepressant Nonresponders with Major Depressive Disorder: A Double-Blind, Randomized Clinical Trial." *American Journal of Psychiatry* 167 (2010): 942–48.

Patricio, Patricia, Antonio Mateus-Pinheiro, Martin Iramler, Nuno D. Alves, Ana R. Machado-Santos, Monica Mrais, Joana S. Correia, Michal Korostynki, Marcin Piechota, Rainer Stoffel, Johanes Beckers, Joao M. Bessa, Osborne F. X. Almeida, Nuno Sousa, and Luisa Pinto. "Differential and Converging Molecular Mechanism of Antidepressants' Action in the Hippocampal Dentate Gyrus." *Neuropsychopharmacology* 40 (2015): 339–49.

Pennix, Brenda W. J., Jack M. Guralnik, Luigi Ferrucci, Eleanor M. Simonsick, Dorly J. H. Deeg, and Robert B. Wallace. "Depressive Symptoms and Physical Decline in Community-Dwelling Older Adults." *Journal of the American Medical Association* 279 (1998): 1720–26.

Pinquart, M., and P. R. Duberstein. "Depression and Cancer Mortality: A Meta-Analysis." *Psychological Medicine* 40 (2010): 1797–1810.

Pirl, William F., Joseph A. Greer, Lara Traeger, Vicki Jackson, Inga T. Lennes, Emily R. Gallagher, Pedro Perz-Cruz, Rebecca S. Heist, and Jennifer S. Temel. "Depression and Survival in Metastatic Non-Small-Cell Lung Cancer: Effects of Early Palliative Care." *Journal of Clinical Oncology* 30 (2012): 1310–15.

Pirmohamed, Munir, Sally James, Shaun Meakin, Chris Green, Andrew K. Scott, Thomas J. Walley, Keith Farrar, B. Kevin Park, and Alasdair M. Breckenridge. "Adverse Drug Reactions as Cause of Admission to Hospital: Prospective Analysis of 18,820 Patients." *British Medical Journal* 329 (2004): 15–19.

Porsteinsson, Anton, and Inga M. Antonsdottir. "Depression and Risk of Dementia: Exploring the Interface." *Journal of Clinical Psychiatry* 74 (2013): 1262–63.

Qian, Jingjing, Linda Simoni-Wastila, Patricia Langenberg, Gail B. Rattinger, Ilene H. Zuckerman, Susan Lehmann, and Michael Terrin. "Effects of Depression Diagnosis and Antidepressant Treatment on Mortality in Medicare Beneficiaries with Chronic Obstructive Pulmonary Disease." *Journal of the American Geriatrics Society* 61 (2013): 754–61.

Quach, Lien, Frances M. Yang, Sarah D. Berry, Elizabeth Newton, Richard N. Jones, Jeffrey A. Burr, and Lewis A. Lipsitz. "Depression, Antidepressants, and Falls among Community-Dwelling Elderly People: The MOBILIZE Boston Study." *Journals of Gerontology: A Biological Science Medical Science* 68 (2013): 1575–81.

Raichle, Katherine A., Joan M. Romano, and Mark P. Jensen. "Partner Responses to Patient Pain and Well Behaviors and Their Relationship to Patient Pain Behavior, Functioning, and Depression." *Pain* 152 (2011): 82–88.

Reich, Michel. "Depression and Cancer: Recent Data on Clinical Issues, Research Challenges, and Treatment Approaches." *Current Opinion in Oncology* 20 (2008): 353–59.

Reid, M. Carrington, Christianna S. Williams, John Concato, Mary E. Tinetti, and Thomas M. Gill. "Depressive Symptoms as a Risk Factor for Disabling Back Pain in Community-Dwelling Older Persons." *Journal of the American Geriatrics Society* 51 (2003): 1710–17.

Reynolds, Charles F., III, Ellen Frank, Mary Amanda Dew, Patricia Houck, Mark Miller, Sati Mazumdar, James M. Perel, and David J. Kupfer. "Treatment of 70+-Year-Olds with Recurrent Major Depression: Excellent Short-Term but Brittle Long-Term Response." *American Journal of Geriatric Psychiatry* 7 (1999): 64–69.

Reynolds, Charles F., III, Ellen Frank, Patricia R. Houck, Sati Mazumbar, Mary Amanda Dew, Cleon Cornes, Daniel J. Buysse, Amy Begley, and David J. Kupfer. "Which Elderly Patients with Remitted Depression Remain Well with Continued Interpersonal Psychotherapy after Discontinuation of Antidepressant Medication?" *American Journal of Psychiatry* 154 (1997): 958–62.

Roberts, Robert E., George A. Kaplan, Sarah J. Shema, and William J. Strawbridge. "Does Growing Old Increase the Risk for Depression?" *American Journal of Psychiatry* 154 (1997): 1384–90.

Rohrbaugh, Robert M., Alan P. Siegal, and Earl L. Giller. "Irritability as a Symptom of Depression in the Elderly." *Journal of the American Geriatrics Society* 1988 (36): 736–38.

Romanelli, Jeanine, James A. Fauerbach, David E. Bush, and Roy C. Ziegelstein. "The Significance of Depression in Older Patients after Myocardial Infarction." *Journal of the American Geriatrics Society* 50 (2002): 817–22.

Roxburgh, Campbell S., and Donald C. McMillan. "Cancer and Systemic Inflammation: Treat the Tumour and Treat the Host." *British Journal of Cancer* 110, no. 6 (2014): 1409–12.

Salzman, Carl, Eileen Wong, and B. Cody Wright. "Drug and ECT Treatment of Depression in the Elderly 1996–2001: A Literature Review." *Biological Psychiatry* 52 (2002): 265–84.

Samuels, Martin. "The Brain-Heart Connection." *Circulation* 116 (2007): 77–84.

Sanmukhani, Jayesh, Vimal Satodia, Jaladhi Trivedi, Tejas Patel, Deepak Tiwari, Bharat Panchal, Ajay Goel, and Chandra Bhanu Tripathi. "Efficacy and Safety of Curcumin in Major Depressive Disorder: A Randomized Controlled Trial." *Phytotherapy Research* 28 (2014): 579–85.

Satlin, Jillian R., Wolfgang Linden, and Melanie J. Phillips. "Depression as a Predictor of Disease Progression and Mortality in Cancer Patients." *Cancer* 115 (2009): 5349–61.

Schroer, Sylvia, Mona Kanaan, Hugh MacPherson, and Joy Adamson. "Acupuncture for Depression: Exploring Model Validity and the Related Issue of Credibility in the Context of Designing a Pragmatic Trial." *CNS Neurosciences and Therapeutics* 18, no. 4 (2012): 318–26.

Sharpe, M., V. Strong, K. Allen, R. Rush, K. Postma, A. Tulloh, P. Maguire, A. House, A. Ramirez, and A. Culi. "Major Depression in Outpatients Attending a Regional Cancer Centre: Screening and Unmet Treatment Needs." *British Journal of Cancer* 90 (2004): 314–20.

Shelton, Richard C. "St. John's Wort (Hypericum Perforatum) in Major Depression." *Journal of Clinical Psychiatry* 70, suppl. 5 (2009): 23–27.

Shen, Cheng-Che, Shih-Jen Tsai, Benjamin Ing-Tiau Kuo, and Albert C. Yang. "Risk of Parkinson Disease after Depression." *Neurology* 81 (2013): 1538–44.

Shriver, Maria. "A Woman's Nation Takes On Alzheimer's." In "The Shriver Report: A Study by Maria Shriver and the Alzheimer's Association." Accessed March 21, 2015. http://www.alz.org.

Sibolt, Gerli, Sami Curtze, Susanna Melkas, Tarja Pohjasvaara, Markku Kaste, Pekka J. Karhunen, Niku K. J. Oksala, Risto Vataja, and Timo Erkinjuntti. "Post-Stroke Depression and Depression-Executive Dysfunction Syndrome Are Associated with Recurrence of Ischemic Stroke." *Cerebrovascular Diseases* 36 (2013): 336–43.

Sigler, Maayanit, Dov Aizenberg, and Abraham Weizman. "Continuation and Maintenance Electroconvulsive Therapy in Elderly Depressed Patients." *International Journal of Geriatric Psychopharmacology* 1, no. 4 (1998): 205–7.

Sloane, Philip D., Mariana Figueiro, and Lauren Cohen. "Light as Therapy for Sleep Disorders and Depression in Older Adults." *Clinical Geriatrics* 16, no. 3 (2008): 25–31.

Sneed, Joel R. "The Vascular Depression Hypothesis: An Update." *American Journal of Geriatric Psychiatry* 19 (2011): 99–103.

Stewart, Jesse, Anthony J. Perkins, and Christopher M. Callahan. "Effect of Collaborative Care for Depression on Risk of Cardiovascular Evens: Data from the IMPACT Randomized Controlled Trial." *Psychosomatic Medicine* 76 (2014): 29–37.

Swanson, David W. "Chronic Pain as a Third Pathologic Emotion." *American Journal of Psychiatry* 141 (1984): 210–14.

Tai-Seale, M., T. McGuire, C. Colenda, D. Rosen, and M. A. Cook. "Two-Minute Mental Health Care for Elderly Patients: Inside Primary Care Visits." *Journal of the American Geriatrics Society* 55 (2007): 1903–11.

Taraz, Mohammad, Saeideh Taraz, and Simin Dashti-Khavidaki. "Association between Depression and Inflammatory/Anti-inflammatory Cytokines in Chronic Kidney Disease and End-Stage Renal Disease Patients: A Review of Literature." *Hemodialysis International* 19 (2015): 11–22.

Tateno, Amane, Mahito Kimura, and Robert Robertson. "Phenomenological Characteristics of Poststroke Depression." *American Journal of Geriatric Psychiatry* 10 (2002): 575–82.

Thomas, Alan. "Is Depression Really Different in Older People?" *International Psychogeriatrics* 25, no. 11 (November 2013): 1739–42. doi: 101017/S1041610213001038.

Thompson, Larry W., David W. Coon, Dolores Gallagher-Thompson, Barbara Sommer, and Diana Koin. "Comparison of Desipramine and Cognitive/Behavioral Therapy in the Treatment of Elderly Outpatients with Mild-to-Moderate Depression." *American Journal of Geriatric Psychiatry* 9 (2001): 225–40.

Tomac, Tracy A., Teresa A. Rummans, Thomas S. Pileggi, and Hongzhe Li. "Safety and Efficacy of Electroconvulsive Therapy in Patients over Age 85." *American Journal of Geriatric Psychiatry* 5 (1997): 126–30.

Turk, Dennis C., Akiko Okifuji, and Lisa Scharff. "Chronic Pain and Depression: Role of Perceived Impact and Perceived Control in Different Age Cohorts." *Pain* 61 (1995): 93–101.

Turk, Dennis C., and Peter Salovey. "Chronic Pain as a Variant of Depressive Disease." *Journal of Nervous and Mental Disease* 172 (1984): 398–407.

van Gool, Coen H., Ertrudis I. J. Kempen, Brenda W. J. H. Penninx, Dorly J. H. Deeg, Aartjan T. F. Beekman, and Jacques T. M. van Eljk. "Relationship between Changes in Depressive Symptoms and Unhealthy Lifestyles in Late Middle Aged and Older Persons: Results from the Longitudinal Aging Study Amsterdam." *Age and Ageing* 32 (2003): 81–87.

van Haastregt, Jolanda C. M., G. A. Rixt Zilstra, Erik van Rossum, Jacques Th. M. van Eijk, and Gertrudis I. J. M. Kempen. "Feelings of Anxiety and Symptoms of Depression in Community-Living Older Persons Who Avoid Activity for Fear of Falling." *American Journal of Geriatric Psychiatry* 16 (2008): 186–93.

Velly, Ana Miriam, John O. Look, Charles Carlson, Patricia A. Lenton, Wenjun Kang, Christina A. Holcroft, and James R. Fricton. "The Effect of Catastrophizing and Depression on Chronic Pain: A Prospective Cohort Study of Temporomandibular Muscle and Joint Pain Disorders." *Pain* 152 (2011): 2377–83.

Verhoeven, Josine E., Dóra Révész, E. S. Epel, J. Lin, Owen M. Wolkowitz, and B. W. J. H. Penninx. "Major Depressive Disorder and Accelerated Cellular Aging: Results from a Large Psychiatric Cohort Study." *Molecular Psychiatry* 19, no. 8 (August 2014): 895–901. Accessed November 12, 2013. doi: 10.1038/mp.2013.151.

Viamontes, George I., and Charles B. Nemeroff. "The Physiologic Effect of Mental Processes on Major Body Systems." *Psychiatric Annals* 40 (2010): 367–80.

Wayne, Peter M., Jacquelyn N. Walsh, Ruth E. Taylor-Piliai, Rebecca Erwin Wells, Kathryn V. Papp, Nancy J. Donovan, and Gloria Y. Yeh. "Effect of Tai Chi on Cognitive Performance in Older Adults: Systematic Review and Meta-Analysis." *Journal of the American Geriatrics Society* 62 (2014): 25–39.

Weintraub, Daniel, and Paul E. Ruskin. "Posttraumatic Stress Disorder in the Elderly: A Review." *Harvard Review of Psychiatry* 7 (1999): 144–52.

Whooly, Mary A., Peter de Jonge, Eric Vittinghoff, Christian Otte, Rudolf Moos, Robert Carney, Sadia Ali, Sunaina Dowray, Beeya Na, Mitchell D. Feldman, Nelson B. Schiller, and Warrren S. Browner. "Depressive Symptoms, Health Behaviors, and Risk of Cardiovascular Events in Patients with Coronary Heart Disease." *Journal of the American Medical Association* 300 (2008): 2379–88.

Wittstein, Ilan S., David R. Thiemann, Joao A. C. Lima, Kenneth L. Baughman, Steven P. Schulman, Gary Gerstenblith, Katherine C. Wu, Jeffrey J. Rade, Trinity J. Bivalqua, and Hunter C. Champion. "Neurohumoral Features of Myocardia Stunning Due to Sudden Emotional Stress." *New England Journal of Medicine* 352 (2005): 539–48.

Wolkowitz, Owen M., Victor I. Reus, and Synthia H. Mellon. "Of Sound Mind and Body: Depression, Disease, and Accelerated Aging." *Dialogues in Clinical Neuroscience* 13 (2011): 25–39.

World Health Association. "Cancer: Fact Sheet." Last updated February 2015. Accessed February 27, 2015. http://www.who.int.

Wu, Junmei, Albert S. Yeung, Rosa Schnyer, Yunfei Wang, and David Mischoulon. "Acupuncture for Depression: A Review of Clinical Applications," *Canadian Journal of Psychiatry* 57, no. 7 (2012): 397–405.

Yang, Yang. "Social Inequalities in Happiness in the United States, 1972 to 2004: An Age-Period-Cohort Analysis." *American Sociological Review* 73 (2008): 204–26.

Yohannes, Abebaw M., Martin Connolly, and Robert C. Baldwin. "A Feasibility Study of Antidepressant Drug Therapy in Depressed Elderly Patients with Chronic Obstructive Pulmonary Disease." *International Journal of Geriatric Psychiatry* 16 (2001): 451–54.

Zalai, Dora, Lilla Szeifert, and Marta Novak. "Psychological Distress and Depression in Patients with Chronic Kidney Disease." *Seminars in Dialysis* 4 (2012): 428–38.

Zautra, Alex J., Mary C. David, and John W. Reich. "Comparison of Cognitive Behavioral and Mindfulness Meditation Interventions on Adaptation to Rheumatoid Arthritis for Patients With and Without History of Recurrent Depression." *Journal of Consulting and Clinical Psychology* 76 (2008): 408–21.

Zesiewicz, Theresa, Michael Gold, Ganesh Chari, and Robert Hauser. "Current Issues in Depression in Parkinson's Disease." *American Journal of Geriatric Psychiatry* 7 (1999): 110–18.

Zilstra, G. A. Rixt, Jolanda C. M. van Haastregt, Erik van Rossum, Jacques Th. M. van Eijk, Lucy Yardley, and Gertrudis I. J. M. Kempen. "Interventions to Reduce Fear of Falling in Community-Living Older People: A Systematic Review." *Journal of the American Geriatrics Society* 55 (2007): 603–15.

Zubenko, George, Wendy Zubenko, Susan McPherson, Eleanor Spoor, Deborah B. Marin, Martin R. Farlow, Glenn E. Smith, Yonas E. Geda, Jeffrey L. Cummings, Ronald C. Petersen, and Trey Sunderland. "A Collaborative Study of the Emergence and Clinical Features of the Major Depression Syndrome of Alzheimer's Disease." *American Journal of Psychiatry* 160 (2003): 857–66.

INDEX

accelerated aging in depression, 76
access to treatment, 265
acupuncture, 239
adjustment disorder with depression. *See*
  Depression
adrenaline, 73
Alzheimer's disease, 36; amyloid levels
  and depression, 168; caregiver stress,
  167; depression as risk factor for, 164;
  depression in, 36; stages, description
  of, 165
anticholinergic effects, 225
antidepressant medication, 208; actions in
  brain, 208, 221; bupropion
  (Wellbutrin), 223; classes of, 221;
  common misconceptions about, 227;
  falls and fractures, risk with, 230;
  mirtazapine (Remeron), 223;
  monoamine oxidase inhibitors
  (MAOIs), 224; rationale for choice,
  226; rationale for use, 220; response
  latency, 250; selective serotonin
  reuptake inhibitors (SSRIs), 222;
  serotonin norepinephrine reuptake
  inhibitors (SNRIs), 223; side effects,
  increased sensitivity to, 249; side
  effects, patient fears of, 201; side
  effects, perspective on, 229; start low,
  go slow approach, 251; strategies for
  use, 227; tricyclic antidepressants
  (TCAs), 224; vilazodone (Viibryd),

223; vortioxetine (Brintellix), 223
apathy, 49
aprosodia, 53
arthritis: arthritis-depression vicious cycle,
  147; definition of, 145; symptom
  overlap with depression, 146;
  treatment of depression in, 148

benzodiazepines: reasons to avoid, 271;
  shortcomings of, 220, 271
bereavement depression. *See* depression
bipolar depression. *See* depression
brain function: circuits, 27; emotions and,
  25; mapping of, 33; networks, 27;
  white matter and, 28
brain-derived neurotrophic factor
  (BDNF), 74; in stroke, 97
brain-heart connection. *See*
  cardiovascular disease
brain imaging, 28; computed tomography
  (CT) and, 28; magnetic resonance
  imaging (MRI) and, 28; positron-
  emission tomography (PET) and, 28;
  single photon emission computed
  tomography (SPECT) and, 28
bupropion (Wellbutrin). *See*
  antidepressants

cancer: definition, 133; depression and
  breast cancer, 137; depression and
  cancer prognosis, 135; depression and